MEDICAL ABBREVIATIONS:

8600 Conveniences at the Expense of Communications and Safety

Sixth Edition

Neil M. Davis, M.S., Pharm.D., FASHP
Professor of Pharmacy, Temple University
  School of Pharmacy, Philadelphia, PA,
Editor-in-Chief, Hospital Pharmacy
Chief Executive Officer, Institute for Safe
  Medication Practices, Inc.

published by

Neil M. Davis Associates
1143 Wright Drive
Huntingdon Valley, PA 19006
Phone (215) 947-1752
FAX (215) 938-1937

Contents

Where an abbreviation contains letters and
numbers, the numbers are not considered
during alphabetizing.

The letter-by-letter (dictionary) system of
alphabetizing is used.

Introduction

isted are 8600 current acronyms, symbols, and other abbreviations and over 13,000 of their possible meanings. This list has been compiled to assist individuals in reading medical records, medically related communications, and prescriptions. The list, although current and comprehensive, represents only a portion of abbreviations in use and their many possible meanings as new ones are being coined every day.

Abbreviations are a convenience, a time saver, a space saver, and a way of avoiding the possibility of misspelling words. However, a price can be paid for their use. Abbreviations are sometimes not understood or are interpreted incorrectly. Their use may lengthen the time needed to train individuals in the health fields, at times delays the patient's care, and occasionally results in patient harm.

The publication of this list of abbreviations is not an endorsement of their legitimacy. It is not a guarantee that the intended meaning has been correctly captured, or an indication that they are in common use. Where uncertainty exists, the one who wrote the abbreviation must be contacted for clarification.

There are many variations in how an abbreviation can be expressed. Anterior-posterior has been written as AP, A.P., ap, and A/P. Since there are few standards and those who use abbreviations do not necessarily follow these standards, this book only shows Anterior-posterior as AP. This is done to make it easier to find the meaning of an abbreviation as all the meanings of AP are listed together. This elimination of unnecessary duplication also keeps the book at a convenient size thus enabling it to be sold at a reasonable price. Lower case letters are used when firm custom dictates as in Ag, Na, mCi, etc.

The Council of Biology Editors (CBE), in their *CBE Style Manual*,[1] lists about 600 abbreviations gathered from 15 internationally recognized authorities and or-

Table 1. Examples of dangerous abbreviations

Problem term	Reason	Suggested term
O.D. for once daily	Interpreted as right eye	Write "once daily"
q.o.d. for every other day	Interpreted as meaning every once a day or read as q.i.d.	Write "every other day"
q.d. for once daily	Read or interpreted as q.i.d.	Write "once daily"
q.n. for every night	Read as every hour	Write "every night," "H.S.," or nightly
q hs for every night	Read as every hour	Use "HS" or "at bedtime"
U for Unit	Read as 0, 4, 6 or cc	Write "unit"
O.J. for orange juice	Read as OD or OS	Write "orange juice"
μg (microgram)	When handwritten, misread as mg	Write "mcg"
sq or sub q for subcutaneous	The q is read as every	Use "subcut"
Chemical symbols	Not understood or misunderstood	Write full name
Lettered abbreviations for drug names or drug protocols	Not understood or misunderstood	Use generic or trade name
Apothecary symbols or terms	Not understood or misunderstood	Use metric system
per os for by mouth	OS read as left eye	Use "by mouth," "orally," or "P.O."
D/C for discharge	Interpreted as discontinue (orders for discharge medications result in premature discontinuance of current medication)	Write "discharge"
T/d for one per day	Read as T.I.D.	Use "once daily"
/ (a slash mark) for with, and, or per	read as a one	use, "and," "with," or "per"

2

ganizations. The majority of these symbols and abbreviations tend to be more scientifically oriented than those which would appear in medical records. In the few situations where the CBE abbreviations differ from what is presented in this book, the CBE abbreviation has been placed in parenthesis after the meaning. As is the practice in the United States, mL has been used rather than ml and the spelling of liter, meter, etc. is used rather than litre and metre, even though ml, litre, and metre are listed in the *CBE Style Manual.*

The abbreviation AP, is listed as meaning doxorubicin and cisplatin. The reason for this apparent disparity is that the official generic names (United States Adopted Names) are shown rather than the trade names Adriamycin® and Platinol®. In the case of LSD, the official name, lysergide, is given, rather than the chemical name, lysergic acid diethylamide. The Latin derivations for older medical and pharmaceutical abbreviations, (TID, *ter in die,* three times daily) may be found in *Remington.*[2]

Healthcare organizations are wisely required by the Joint Commission on Accreditation of Healthcare Organizations to formulate an approved list of abbreviations. Every attempt should be made to restrict this list to common abbreviations that are understood by all health professionals who must work with medical records. There are certain dangerous abbreviations that should not be approved, and a warning should be issued about their use (see Table 1 as well as notes in the text). A second list should also be published containing dangerous abbreviations which were purposely omitted from the approved list. The reasons for their omission should be stated.

Many inherent problems associated with abbreviations contribute to or cause errors. Reports of such errors have been published routinely.[3-5]

Abbreviations and symbols can also easily be misread or interpreted in a manner not intended. For example:

    (1) "HCT250 mg" was intended to mean hydrocortisone 250 mg but was interpreted as hydrochlorothiazide 50 mg (HCTZ50 mg).

(2) Flucytosine was improperly abbreviated as 5 FU causing it to be read as fluorouracil. Flucytosine is abbreviated 5 FC and fluorouracil is 5 FU.

(3) Floxuridine was improperly abbreviated as 5 FU causing it to be read as fluorouracil. Floxuridine is abbreviated FUDR and fluorouracil is 5 FU.

(4) MTX was thought to be mustargen. MTX is methotrexate and mustargen is abbreviated HN_2.

(5) **The abbreviation "U" for unit is the most dangerous one in the book, having caused numerous 10 fold insulin overdoses. The word unit should never be abbreviated.** The handwritten U for unit has been mistaken for a zero, causing tenfold errors. The handwritten U has also been read as the number four, six, and as "cc."

(6) OD meant to signify once daily has caused Lugol's solution to be given in the right eye.

(7) OJ meant to signify orange juice, looked like OS and caused Saturated Solution of Potassium Iodide to be given in the left eye.

Table 2. Example of abbreviations which have several meanings

CPM	= cyclophosphamide; chlorpheniramine maleate; continuous passive motion; continue present management; central pontine myelinolysis; counts per minute; and clinical practice model
PBZ	= phenylbutazone; pyribenzamine; phenoxybenzamine
CPZ	= chlorpromazine; Compazine®
DW	= dextrose in water; distilled water; deionized water
LFD	= lactose-free diet; low fat diet; and low fiber diet
MS	= morphine sulfate; multiple sclerosis; mitral stenosis; musculoskeletal; medical student; minimal support; muscle strength; mental status; milk shake; mitral sound; and morning stiffness
CF	= cystic fibrosis; Caucasian female; calcium leucovorin (citrovorum factor); complement fixation; cancer-free; cardiac failure; coronary flow; contractile force; cephalothin; Christmas factor; count fingers; and cisplatin and fluorouracil
NBM	= no bowel movement; normal bowel movement; nothing by mouth; normal bone marrow

(8) Na Warfarin (Sodium Warfarin) was read as "No Warfarin."

(9) The abbreviation "s̄" for without has been thought to mean "with" (c̄).

(10) The order for PT, intended to signify a laboratory test order for prothrombin time, resulted in the ordering of a physical therapy consultation.

(11) The abbreviation, "TAB," meant to signify Triple Antibiotic, (a coined name for a hospital sterile topical antibiotic mixture), caused patients to have their wound irrigated with a diet soda.

(12) A slash mark (/) has been mistaken for a one, causing a patient to receive a 100 unit overdose of NPH insulin when the slash was used to separate an order for two insulin doses:

6 units regular insulin/20 units NPH insulin

A prescription could be written with directions as follows: "OD OD OD," to mean one drop in the right eye once daily!

Abbreviations should not be used for drug names as they are particularly dangerous. As previously illustrated, there is the possibility that the writer may, through mental error, confuse two abbreviations and use the wrong one. Similarly, the reader may attribute the wrong meaning to an abbreviation. To further confound the problem, some drug name abbreviations have multiple meanings (see CPM, CPZ and PBZ in table 2). The abbreviation AC has been used for three different cancer chemotherapy combinations to mean, Adriamycin® and either cyclophosphamide, carmustine, or cisplatin. Beside causing medication errors and incorrect interpretation of medical records, abbreviations can create problems because treatment is delayed while a health professional seeks clarification for the meaning of the abbreviation used. Abbreviations should not be used to designate drugs or combinations of drugs.

Certain abbreviations in the book are followed by a warning, "this is a dangerous abbreviation." This warning could be placed after most abbreviations, but was reserved for situations where errors have been published because these abbreviations were used or where the meaning is critical and not likely to be known. Such warning statements should also appear after every abbreviation for a drug or drug combination.

Abbreviations for medical facility names create problems as they are usually not recognized by the reader in another geographic area. A clue to the fact that one is dealing with such an abbreviation is when it ends with MC, for Medical Center; MH, for Memorial Hospital; CH, for Community Hospital; UH, for University Hospital; and H, for Hospital.

When an abbreviation can not be found in the book or when the listed meaning(s) do not make sense, there is a possibility that the abbreviation has been misread. As an example, a reader could not find the meaning of HHTS. On closer examination it really was +HTS, not HHTS.

Listed in the rear of the book is a table of normal laboratory values. Both the conventional and international values are listed. Each laboratory publishes a list of its normal values. These local lists should be reviewed to see if there are significant differences.

An examination of the following list is a testimonial to the problems and dangers associated with most undefined abbreviations.

The assistance of Aphirudee Poshakrishma Hemachudha, former teaching assistant, Temple University School of Pharmacy, Philadelphia, PA; Michael R. Cohen, Ann Sandt Kishbaugh, Merchantville, NJ; Evelyn Canizares and all the others that helped is gratefully acknowledged.

6

A

A accommodation
age
alive
ambulatory
angioplasty
anterior
anxiety
apical
arterial
artery
Asian
assessment
(a at
(a) axillary temperature
ā before
A_2 aortic second sound
A250 5% albumin 250 mL
A1000 5% albumin 1000 mL
A II angiotensin II
AA acetic acid
achievement age
active assistive
acute asthma
Alcoholics Anonymous
alcohol abuse
alveolar-arterial gradient
amino acid
anti-aerobic
antiarrhythmic agent
aortic aneurysm
aplastic anemia
arm ankle (pulse ratio)
ascending aorta
audiologic assessment
authorized absence
automobile accident
cytarabine and
doxorubicin
aa of each
A&A arthroscopy and
arthrotomy
awake and aware
AAA abdominal aortic
aneurysmectomy
(aneurysm)

acute anxiety attack
aromatic amino acids
AAC Adrenalin®, atropine, and
cocaine
antimicrobial
agent-associated colitis
AACG acute angle closure
glaucoma
AAD acid-ash diet
antibiotic-associated
diarrhea
[A-a]Do$_2$ alveolar-arterial oxygen
tension gradient
AAE active assistance exercise
acute allergic encephalitis
A/AEX active assistive exercise
AAG alpha-1-acid glycoprotein
AAL anterior axillary line
AAM amino acid mixture
AAMS acute aseptic meningitis
syndrome
AAN analgesic abuse
nephropathy
analgesic-associated
nephropathy
attending's admission
notes
AAO alert, awake, & oriented
AAO × 3 awake and oriented to
time, place, and person
AAOC antacid of choice
AAP assessment adjustment
pass
AAPC antibiotic-acquired
pseudomembranous
colitis
AAPMC antibiotic-associated
pseudomembranous
colitis
AAR antigen-antiglobulin
reaction
AAROM active assistive range of
motion
AAS acute abdominal series
androgenic-anabolic
steroid
aortic arch syndrome
atlantoaxis subluxation
atypical absence seizure

AASCRN	amino acid screen		ABE	acute bacterial endocarditis
AAT	alpha-antitrypsin			adult basic education
	at all times			botulism equine trivalent antitoxin
	atypical antibody titer			
A_1AT	alpha$_1$-antitrypsin		ABEP	auditory brain stem-evoked potentials
A_1AT-P_i	alpha$_1$-antitrypsin (phenotyping)		ABF	aortobifemoral (bypass)
AAU	acute anterior uveitis		ABG	air/bone gap
AAV	adeno-associated virus			aortoiliac bypass graft
AAVV	accumulated alveolar ventilatory volume			arterial blood gases
				axiobuccogingival
AB	abortion		ABH	Ativan®, Benadryl®, and Haldol®
	Ace® bandage			
	antibiotic		ABI	atherothrombotic brain infarction
	antibody			
	Aphasia Battery		ABID	antibody identification
	apical beat		A Big	atrial bigeminy
	armboard		ABK	aphakic bullous keratopathy
A/B	acid-base ratio			
	apnea/bradycardia		ABL	allograft bound lymphocytes
A > B	air greater than bone (conduction)			
			ABLB	alternate binaural loudness balance
A & B	apnea and bradycardia			
ABC	abbreviated blood count		A/B Mods	apnea/bradycardia moderate stimulation
	absolute band counts			
	absolute basophil count		A/B MS	apnea/bradycardia mild stimulation
	aneurysmal bone cyst			
	antigen binding capacity		ABMT	autologous bone marrow transplantation
	apnea, bradycardia, and cyanosis			
			ABN	abnormality(ies)
	argon beam coagulator		A.B.N.M.	American Board of Nuclear Medicine
	aspiration, biopsy and cytology			
			abnor.	abnormal
	artificial beta cells		ABO	blood group system (A, AB, B, and O)
	avidin-biotin complex			
ABCDE	botulism toxoid pentavalent		ABP	arterial blood pressure
			ABPA	allergic bronchopulmo-nary aspergillosis
ABD	after bronchodilator			
ABd	plain gauze dressing, type of		ABPM	ambulatory blood pressure monitoring
Abd	abdomen		ABR	absolute bed rest
	abdominal			auditory brain (evoked) responses
	abductor			
ABDCT	atrial bolus dynamic computer tomography		ABS	absent
				absorbed
ABD GR	abdominal girth			absorption
ABD PB	abductor pollicis brevis			Accuchek® blood sugar
ABD PL	abductor pollicis longus			acute brain syndrome

	admitting blood sugar	AcCoA	acetyl-coenzyme A
	at bedside	ACCR	amylase creatinine
A/B SS	apnea/bradycardia		clearance ratio
	self-stimulation	ACCU	acute coronary care unit
ABT	aminopyrine breath test	ACCU✔	Accuchek® (blood
ABVD	Adriamycin®, bleomycin,		glucose monitoring)
	vinblastine, and	ACD	absolute cardiac dullness
	dacarbazine (DTIC)		acid-citrate-dextrose
ABW	actual body weight		allergic contact dermatitis
ABx	antibiotics		anemia of chronic disease
AC	abdominal circumference		anterior chamber diameter
	acetate		anterior chest diameter
	acromioclavicular		dactinomycin
	acute	ACDDS	Alcoholism/Chemical
	air conditioned		Dependency
	air conduction		Detoxification Service
	anchored catheter	ACDK	acquired cystic disease of
	antecubital		the kidney
	anticoagulant	ACDs	anticonvulsant drugs
	assist control	ACE	angiotensin-converting
	activated charcoal		enzyme
	before meals	ACEI	angiotensin-converting
A/C	anterior chamber of the		enzyme inhibitor
	eye	ACF	accessory clinical findings
	assist/control		acute care facility
5-AC	azacitidine		anterior cervical fusion
ACA	acyclovir	ACHES	abdominal pain, chest
	adenocarcinoma		pain, headache, eye
	aminocaproic acid		problems, and severe
	anterior cerebral artery		leg pains (early danger
	anterior communicating		signs of oral
	artery		contraceptive adverse
	anticanalicular antibodies		effects)
AC/A	accommodation	ACG	angiocardiography
	convergence–accommo-	ACH	adrenal cortical hormone
	dation (ratio)		aftercoming head
ACB	alveolar-capillary block		arm girth, chest depth,
	antibody-coated bacteria		and hip width
	before breakfast	ACh	acetylcholine
AC & BC	air and bone conduction	AChE	acetylcholinesterase
ACBE	air contrast barium enema	AC & HS	before meals and at
ACC	accident		bedtime
	accommodation	ACI	adrenal cortical
	adenoid cystic carcinomas		insufficiency
	administrative control		aftercare instructions
	center	ACJ	acromioclavicular joint
	ambulatory care center	A/CK	Accuchek®
	amylase creatinine	ACL	anterior cruciate ligament
	clearance	aCL	anticardiolipin (antibody)

ACLR	anterior cruciate ligament repair		air dyne
ACLS	advanced cardiac life support		alternating days (this is a dangerous abbreviation)
ACME	aphakic cystoid macular edema		Alzheimer's disease
			axis deviation
ACMV	assist-controlled mechanical ventilation	A&D	right ear
			alcohol and drug
ACN	acute conditioned neurosis		ascending and descending
A COMM A	anterior communicating artery		vitamins A and D
		ADA	adenosine deaminase
ACP	acid phosphatase		American Diabetes Association
ACPA	anticytoplasmic antibodies		anterior descending artery
AC-PH	acid phosphatase	ADAM	adjustment disorder with anxious mood
ACPP	adrenocorticopolypeptide		
ACPP PF	acid phosphatase prostatic fluid	ADAU	adolescent drug abuse unit
		ADC	Aid to Dependent Children
ACR	adenomatosis of the colon and rectum		anxiety disorder clinic
	anterior chamber reformation	ADCC	antibody-dependent cellular cytotoxicity
	anticonstipation regimen	ADD	adduction
ACS	American Cancer Society		attention deficit disorder
	anodal-closing sound		average daily dose
	before supper	ADDH	attention deficit disorder with hyperactivity
ACSL	automatic computerized solvent litholysis	ADDL	additional
ACSVBG	aortocoronary saphenous vein bypass graft	ADDM	adjustment disorder with depressed mood
ACSW	Academy of Certified Social Workers	ADDP	adductor pollicis
		ADDU	alcohol and drug dependence unit
ACT	activated clotting time	ADE	acute disseminated encephalitis
	allergen challenge test		
	anticoagulant therapy	ADEM	acute disseminating encephalomyelitis
ACT-D	dactinomycin		
Act Ex	active exercise	AEDP	assisted end diastolic pressure
ACTG	AIDS Clinical Trial Group		
		ADFU	agar diffusion for fungus
ACTH	corticotropin (adrenocorticotrophic hormone)	ADG	atrial diastolic gallop
		ADH	antidiuretic hormone
ACTSEB	anterior chamber tube shunt encircling band	ADHD	attention-deficit hyperactivity disorder
ACV	acyclovir	ADI	allowable daily intake
	atrial/carotid/ventricular	A-DIC	doxorubicin and dacarbazine
ACVD	acute cardiovascular disease		
		ADL	activities of daily living
AD	accident dispensary	*ad lib*	as desired
	admitting diagnosis		at liberty

10

ADM	admission		A&E	accident and emergency
	doxorubicin			(department)
ADME	absorption, distribution,		AEA	above elbow amputation
	metabolism, and		AEB	as evidenced by
	excretion			atrial ectopic beat
Ad-OAP	doxorubicin, vincristine,		AEC	at earliest convenience
	cytarabine, and		AED	antiepileptic drug
	prednisone			automated external
ADOL	adolescent			defibrillator
ADP	arterial demand pacing		AEDP	automated external
	adenosine diphosphate			defibrillator pacemaker
ADPKD	autosomal dominant		AEEU	admission entrance and
	polycystic kidney			evaluation unit
	disease		AEG	air encephalogram
ADQ	abductor digiti quinti			Alcohol Education Group
	adequate		AEM	ambulatory electrogram
ADR	acute dystonic reaction			monitor
	adverse drug reaction		AEP	auditory evoked potential
	doxorubicin		AEq	age equivalent
	(Adriamycin®)		AER	acoustic evoked response
ADRIA	doxorubicin			auditory evoked response
	(Adriamycin®)		Aer. M.	aerosol mask
ADS	admission day surgery		Aer. T.	aerosol tent
	anatomical dead space		AES	anti-embolic stockings
	anonymous donor's sperm		AEs	adverse events
	antibody deficiency		AET	alternating esotropia
	syndrome			atrial ectopic tachycardia
ADSU	ambulatory diagnostic		AF	acid-fast
	surgery unit			afebrile
ADT	alternate-day therapy			amniotic fluid
	anticipate discharge			anterior fontanel
	tomorrow			antifibrinogen
	Auditory Discrimination			aortofemoral
	Test			atrial fibrillation
ADTP	Adolescent Day		AFB	acid-fast bacilli
	Treatment Program			aorto-femoral bypass
	Alcohol Dependence			aspirated foreign body
	Treatment Program		AFBG	aortofemoral bypass graft
A5D5W	alcohol 5%, dextrose 5%		AFC	adult foster care
	in water for injection			air filled cushions
ADX	audiological diagnostic		AFDC	Aid to Family and
AE	above elbow (amputation)			Dependent Children
	accident and emergency		AFE	amniotic fluid
	(department)			embolization
	acute exacerbation		AFEB	afebrile
	air entry		aFGF	acidic fibroblast growth
	antiembolitic			factor
	arm ergometer		AFI	amniotic fluid index
	aryepiglottic (fold)		A fib	atrial fibrillation

AFIP	Armed Forces Institute of Pathology
AFKO	ankle-foot-knee orthosis
AFL	atrial flutter
AFLP	acute fatty liver of pregnancy
AFO	ankle-foot orthosis
AFOF	anterior fontanel–open and flat
AFP	alpha-fetoprotein
	ascending frontal parietal
AFRD	acute febrile respiratory disease
AFV	amniotic fluid volume
AFVSS	afebrile, vital signs stable
AFX	air-fluid exchange
AG	abdominal girth
	aminoglycoside
	anion gap
	antigen
	anti-gravity
	atrial gallop
Ag	silver
A/G	albumin to globulin ratio
AGA	accelerated growth area
	acute gonococcal arthritis
	appropriate for gestational age
	average gestational age
AG/BL	aminoglycoside/beta-lactam
AGD	agar gel diffusion
AGE	acute gastroenteritis
	angle of greatest extension
	irreversible advanced glycosylation end products
AGF	angle of greatest flexion
AGG	agammaglobulinemia
aggl.	agglutination
AGL	acute granulocytic leukemia
A GLAC-TO-LK	alpha galactoside leukocytes
AGN	acute glomerulonephritis
AgNO₃	silver nitrate
AGPT	agar-gel precipitation test
AGS	adrenogenital syndrome

AGTT	abnormal glucose tolerance test
AH	abdominal hysterectomy
	amenorrhea-hyperprolac-tinemia
	antihyaluronidase
A&H	accident and health (insurance)
AHA	acetohydroxamic acid (Lithostat®)
	acquired hemolytic anemia
	autoimmune hemolytic anemia
AHB_c	hepatitis B core antibody
AHC	acute hemorrhagic conjunctivitis
	acute hemorrhagic cystitis
AHD	arteriosclerotic heart disease
	autoimmune hemolytic disease
AHE	acute hemorrhagic encephalomyelitis
AHEC	Area Health Education Center
AHF	antihemophilic factor
AHFS	American Hospital Formulary Service
AHG	antihemophilic globulin
AHGS	acute herpetic gingival stomatitis
AHHD	arteriosclerotic hypertensive heart disease
AHI	apnea/hypopnea index
AHJ	artificial hip joint
AHL	apparent half-life
AHM	ambulatory Holter monitoring
AHN	adenomatous hyperplastic nodule
	Assistant Head Nurse
AHP	acute hemorrhagic pancreatitis
AHS	adaptive hand skills
AHT	alternating hypertropia
	autoantibodies to human thyroglobulin

AI	accidentally incurred	AIN	acute interstitial nephritis
	apical impulse		anal intraepithelial
	allergy index		neoplasia
	aortic insufficiency	AINS	anti-inflammatory
	artificial insemination		non-steroidal
	artificial intelligence	AIOD	aortoiliac occlusive
A & I	Allergy and Immunology		disease
	(department)	AION	anterior ischemic optic
AIA	anti-insulin antibody		neuropathy
	aspirin-induced asthma	AIP	acute infectious
AI-Ab	anti-insulin antibody		polyneuritis
AIBF	anterior interbody fusion		acute intermittent
AICA	anterior inferior cerebellar		porphyria
	artery	AIR	accelerated idioventricular
	anterior inferior		rhythm
	communicating artery	AIS	Abbreviated Injury Score
AICD	automatic implantable		anti-insulin serum
	cardioverter/defibrilla-	AIS/ISS	Abbreviated Injury
	tor		Scale/Injury Severity
AID	acute infectious disease		Score
	artificial insemination	AITP	autoimmune
	donor		thrombocytopenia
	automatic implantable		purpura
	defibrillator	AIU	absolute iodine uptake
AIDH	artificial insemination	AIVR	accelerated idioventricular
	donor husband		rhythm
AIDKS	acquired immune	AJ	ankle jerk
	deficiency syndrome	AJR	abnormal jugular reflex
	with Kaposi's sarcoma	AK	above knee (amputation)
AIDS	acquired immune		actinic keratosis
	deficiency syndrome		artificial kidney
AIE	acute inclusion body	AKA	above-knee amputation
	encephalitis		alcoholic ketoacidosis
AIF	aortic-iliac-femoral		all known allergies
AIH	artificial insemination		also known as
	with husband's sperm	AKS	arthroscopic knee surgery
AIHA	autoimmune hemolytic	AKU	artificial kidney unit
	anemia	AL	acute leukemia
AIHD	acquired immune		argon laser
	hemolytic disease		arterial line
AIIS	anterior inferior iliac		axial length
	spine		left ear
AILD	angioimmunoblastic	ALA	aminolevulinic acid
	lymphadenopathy (with	ALAC	antibiotic-loaded acrylic
	dysproteinemia)		cement
AIMS	Abnormal Involuntary	ALAD	abnormal left axis
	Movement Scale		deviation
	Arthritis Impact	ALARA	as low as reasonably
	Measurement Scales		achievable

ALAT	alanine transaminase (alanine aminotransferase; SGPT)	ALT	alanine transaminase (SGPT) argon laser trabeculoplasty
ALAX	apical long axis	2 alt	every other day (this is a dangerous abbreviation)
Alb	albumin albuterol	ALTB	acute laryngotracheobronchitis
ALC	acute lethal catatonia alcohol alcoholic liver cirrhosis	ALTE	acute life threatening event
	allogeneic lymphocyte cytotoxicity	ALUP	Alupent®
	alternate level of care	ALVAD	abdominal left ventricular assist device
	alternate lifestyle checklist	ALWMI	anterolateral wall myocardial infarct
ALC R	alcohol rub		
ALD	adrenoleukodystrophy alcoholic liver disease aldolase	AM	adult male amalgam anovulatory menstruation
ALDOST	aldosterone		morning (a.m.) myopic astigmatism
ALFT	abnormal liver function tests	AMA	against medical advice American Medical Association antimitochondrial antibody
ALG	antilymphoblast globulin antilymphocyte globulin		
ALI	argon laser iridotomy		
A-line	arterial catheter		
alk	alkaline	AMAD	morning admission
ALK ISO	alkaline phosphatase isoenzymes	AMAG	adrenal medullary autograft
ALK-P	alkaline phosphatase	AMAL	amalgam
ALL	acute lymphoblastic leukemia	AMAP	as much as possible
	acute lymphocytic leukemia	AMAT	anti-malignant antibody test
	allergy	A-MAT	amorphous material
ALM	acral lentiginous melanoma	AMB	ambulate ambulatory amphotericin B as manifested by
ALMI	anterolateral myocardial infarction		
ALN	anterior lymph node	AMBER	advanced multiple beam equalization radiography
Al(OH)₃	aluminum hydroxide		
ALP	argon laser photocoagulation	AMC	arm muscle circumference
	Alupent®	AM/CR	amylase to creatinine ratio
ALPZ	alprazolam	AMD	age-related macular degeneration dactinomycin (actinomycin D) methyldopa (alpha methyldopa)
ALRI	anterolateral rotary instability		
ALS	acute lateral sclerosis advanced life support amyotrophic lateral sclerosis		
		AME	agreed medical examination

AMegL	acute megokaryoblastic leukemia	amt.	amount
AMES-LAN	American sign language	AMTS	Abbreviated Mental Test Score
AMF	aerobic metabolism facilitator	AMU	accessory-muscle use
	autocrine motility factor	AMV	alveolar minute ventilation
AMG	acoustic myography		assisted mechanical ventilation
	aminoglycoside	AMY	amylase
AMI	acute myocardial infarction	AN	anorexia nervosa
	amitriptyline		Associate Nurse
AML	acute myelogenous leukemia	ANA	antinuclear antibody
	angiomyolipoma	ANAD	anorexia nervosa and associated disorders
AMM	agnogenic myeloid metaplasia	ANA SWAB	anaerobic swab
AMML	acute myelomonocytic leukemia	ANC	absolute neutrophil count
		ANCA	antineutrophil cytoplasmic antibody
AMMOL	acute myelomonoblastic leukemia	anch	anchored
AMN	adrenomyeloneuropathy	ANCOVA	analysis of covariance
amnio	amniocentesis	AND	anterior nasal discharge
AMN SC	amniotic fluid scan	ANDA	Abbreviated New Drug Application
AMOL	acute monoblastic leukemia	anes	anesthesia
AMP	adenosine monophosphate	ANF	antinuclear factor
	ampicillin		atrial natriuretic factor
	ampul	ANG	angiogram
	amputation	ANISO	anisocytosis
A-M pr	Austin-Moore prosthesis	ANLL	acute nonlymphoblastic leukemia
AMPT	metyrosine (alphamethylpara tyrosine)	ANOVA	analysis of variance
AMR	alternating motor rates	ANP	atrial natriuretic peptide (anaritide acetate)
AMS	acute mountain sickness	ANS	answer
	aggravated in military service		autonomic nervous system
	altered mental status	ANT	anterior
	amylase		enpheptin (2-amino-5-nitrothiazol)
	auditory memory span	ante	before
m-AMSA	amsacrine (acridinyl anisidide)	ANTI A:AGT	anti blood group A antiglobulin test
AMSIT	portion of the mental status examination: A—appearance, M—mood, S—sensorium, I—intelligence, T—thought process	Anti bx	antibiotic
		ant sag D	anterior sagittal diameter
		ANTU	alpha naphthylthiourea
		ANUG	acute necrotizing ulcerative gingivitis
		ANX	anxiety
			anxious

AO	Agent Orange		apical pulse
	anterior oblique		appendectomy
	aorta		appendicitis
	aortic opening		atrial pacing
	plate, screw (orthopedics)		attending physician
	right ear		doxorubicin and cisplatin
A & O	alert and oriented	A&P	active and present
A&O × 3	awake and oriented to		anterior and posterior
	person, place, and time		assessment and plans
A&O × 4	awake and oriented to		auscultation and
	person, place, time,		percussion
	and date	A/P	ascites/plasma ratio
AOAP	as often as possible	$A_2 > P_2$	second aortic sound
AOB	alcohol on breath		greater than second
AOC	anode opening contraction		pulmonic sound
	antacid of choice	APACHE	Acute Physiology and
	area of concern		Chronic Health
AOCD	anemia of chronic disease		Evaluation
AOD	alleged onset date	APAD	anterior-posterior
	arterial occlusive disease		abdominal diameter
	Assistant-Officer-of-the-	APAG	antipseudomonal
	Day		aminoglycosidic
AODA	alcohol and other drug		penicillin
	abuse	APAP	acetaminophen (N
AODM	adult onset diabetes		acetyl-para-
	mellitus		aminophenol)
ao-il	aorta-iliac	APB	abductor pollicis brevis
AOM	acute otitis media		atrial premature beat
	alternatives of	APC	adenoidal-pharyngeal-
	management		conjunctival
AONAD	alert, oriented, and no		adenomatous polyposis of
	acute distress		the colon and rectum
AOO	continuous arterial		antigen-presenting cell
	asynchronous pacing		aspirin, phenacetin, and
AOP	aortic pressure		caffeine
AOR	Alvarado Orthopedic		atrial premature
	Research		contraction
	at own risk		autologous packed cells
AOS	ambulatory outpatient	APCD	adult polycystic disease
	surgery	APD	action potential duration
	antibiotic order sheet		afferent pupillary defect
AOSD	adult-onset Still's disease		pamidronate disodium
AP	acute pancreatitis		(aminohydroxypropyli-
	aerosol pentamidine		dene diphosphate)
	alkaline phosphatase		anterior-posterior diameter
	angina pectoris		atrial premature
	antepartum		depolarization
	anterior-posterior (x-ray)		automated peritoneal
	arterial pressure		dialysis

APDC	Anxiety and Panic Disorder Clinic	APR	abdominoperineal resection
APE	absolute prediction error	APRV	airway pressure release ventilation
	acute psychotic episode		
	acute pulmonary edema	APS	Acute Physiology Scoring (system)
APG	Apgar (score)		
APGAR	appearance (color), pulse (heart rate), grimace (reflex irritability), activity (muscle tone), and respiration (score reflecting condition of newborn)		adult protective services
			Adult Psychiatric Service
		APSAC	anistreplase (anisoylated plasminogen streptokinase activator complex)
		APSD	Alzheimer's presenile dementia
APH	adult psychiatric hospital		
	alcohol-positive history	APSP	assisted peak systolic pressure
	antepartum hemorrhage		
APIVR	artificial pacemaker-induced ventricular rhythm	aPTT	activated partial thromboplastin time
		APU	ambulatory procedure unit
APKD	adult polycystic kidney disease		antepartum unit
		APUD	amine precursor uptake and decarboxylation
	adult-onset polycystic kidney disease		
		APVC	partial anomalous pulmonary venous connection
APL	abductor pollicis longus		
	accelerated painless labor		
	acute promyelocytic leukemia	APVR	aortic pulmonary valve replacement
	anterior pituitary-like (hormone)	aq	water
		AQ	accomplishment quotient
	chorionic gonadotropin	aq dest	distilled water
AP & L	anteroposterior and lateral	A quad	atrial quadragemimy
APMPPE	acute posterior multifocal placoid pigment epitheliopathy	AR	acoustic reflex
			active resistance
			airway resistance
APN	acute pyelonephritis		alcohol related
APO	adverse patient occurrence		aortic regurgitation
	apolipoprotein A-1		aural rehabilitation
	doxorubicin, prednisone, and vincristine		autorefractor
		Ar	argon
apo E	apolipoprotein E	A&R	adenoidectomy with radium
APPG	aqueous procaine penicillin G (dangerous terminology; for intramuscular use only, write as penicillin G procaine)		
			advised and released
		A-R	apical-radial (pulses)
		ARA	adenosine regulating agent
		ARA-A	vidarabine
appr.	approximate	ARA-AC	fazarabine
appt.	appointment	ARA-C	cytarabine
APPY	appendectomy	ARB	any reliable brand

ARBOR	arthropod-borne virus		Achilles (tendon) reflex test
ARBOW	artificial rupture of bag of water		acoustic reflex threshold(s)
ARC	abnormal retinal correspondence		assessment, review, and treatment
	anomalous retinal correspondence		arterial
	AIDS related complex		automated reagin test (for syphilis)
	American Red Cross		
ARCBS	American Red Cross Blood Services	ARTIC	articulation
		Art T	art therapy
ARD	acute respiratory disease	ARU	alcohol rehabilitation unit
	adult respiratory distress	ARV	AIDS related virus
	antibiotic removal device	ARW	Accredited Rehabilitation Worker
	antibiotic retrieval device		
	aphakic retinal detachment	ARWY	airway
		AS	activated sleep
ARDS	adult respiratory distress syndrome		anal sphincter
			ankylosing spondylitis
ARE	active-resistive exercises		anterior synechia
ARF	acute renal failure		aortic stenosis
	acute respiratory failure		atherosclerosis
	acute rheumatic fever		doctor called through answering service
ARG	arginine		
ARI	acute renal insufficiency		atropine sulfate
	aldose reductase inhibitor		AutoSuture®
ARLD	alcohol related liver disease		left ear
		ASA	aspirin (acetylsalicylic acid)
ARM	anxiety reaction, mild		
	artificial rupture of membranes		American Society of Anesthesiologists
ARMD	age-related macular degeneration		argininosuccinate
		ASA I	Healthy patient with localized pathological process
ARMS	amplification refractory mutation system		
ARN	acute retinal necrosis	ASA II	A patient with mild to moderate systemic disease
AROM	active range of motion		
	artifical rupture of membranes	ASA III	A patient with severe systemic disease limiting activity but not incapacitating
ARP	absolute refractory period		
	alcohol rehabilitation program		
arr	arrive	ASA IV	A patient with incapacitating systemic disease
A.R.R.T.	American Registry of Radiologic Technologists		
		ASA V	Moribund patient not expected to live.
ARS	antirabies serum		(These are American Society of
ART	Accredited Record Technician		

	Anesthesiologists' patient classifications. Emergency operations are designated by "E" after the classification.)	ASHD	arteriosclerotic heart disease
5-ASA	mesalamine (5-aminosalicylic acid) (this is a dangerous abbreviation as it is mistaken for five aspirin tablets)	ASI	Anxiety Status Inventory
		ASIS	anterior superior iliac spine
		ASK	antistreptokinase
		ASL	antistreptolysin (titer)
		ASLO	antistreptolysin-O
ASAA	acquired severe aplastic anemia	ASLV	avian sarcoma and leukosis virus (Rous virus)
ASACL	American Society of Anesthesiologists Classification	AsM	myopic astigmatism
		ASMA	anti-smooth muscle antibody
AS/AI	aortic stenosis/aortic insufficiency	ASMI	anteroseptal myocardial infarction
A's and B's	apnea and bradycardia	ASO	aldicarb sulfoxide antistreptolysin-O titer arteriosclerosis obliterans automatic stop order
ASAP	as soon as possible		
ASAT	aspartate transaminase (aspartate aminotransferase) (SGOT)	ASOT	antistreptolysin-O titer
		ASP	acute suppurative parotitis acute symmetric polyarthritis asparaginase aspartic acid
ASB	anesthesia standby asymptomatic bacteriuria		
ASC	altered state of consciousness		
	ambulatory surgery center anterior subcapsular cataract	ASPVD	arteriosclerotic peripheral vascular disease
		ASR	automatic speech recognition
	antimony sulfur colloid ascorbic acid	ASS	anterior superior supine assessment
ASCVD	arteriosclerotic cardiovascular disease	asst	assistant
ASD	atrial septal defect aldosterone secretion defect	AST	Aphasia Screening Test aspartate transaminase (SGOT) astemizole astigmatism
ASD I	atrial septal defect, primum		
		AS TOL	as tolerated
ASD II	atrial septal defect, secundum	ASTIG	astigmatism
		ASTZ	antistreptozyme test
ASDH	acute subdural hematoma	ASU	acute stroke unit ambulatory surgical unit
ASE	acute stress erosion		
ASF	anterior spinal fusion	ASV	antisnake venom
ASH	asymmetric septal hypertrophy	ASVD	arteriosclerotic vessel disease
AsH	hypermetropic astigmatism	ASYM	asymmetric (al)
		AT	activity therapy (therapist) antithrombin

	applanation tonometry	ATR	Achilles tendon reflex
	atraumatic		atrial
AT 10	dihydrotachysterol		atropine
ATB	antibiotic	atr fib	atrial fibrillation
ATC	aerosol treatment chamber	ATRO	atropine
	alcoholism therapy classes	ATU	alcohol treatment unit
	around the clock	ATS	antitetanic serum (tetanus
	Arthritis Treatment Center		antitoxin)
ATD	antithyroid drug(s)		anxiety tension state
	asphyxiating thoracic	ATSO4	atropine sulfate
	dystrophy	ATT	arginine tolerance test
	autoimmune thyroid	at. wt	atomic weight
	disease	AU	allergenic units
ATE	adipose tissue extraction		both ears
At Fib	atrial fibrillation	Au	gold
AT III FUN	antithrombin III	198Au	radioactive gold
	functional	AUB	abnormal uterine bleeding
ATG	antithymocyte globulin	AUC	area under the curve
ATHR	angina threshold heart	AUCt	area under the curve to
	rate		last time point
ATI	Abdominal Trauma Index	AUD	auditory comprehension
ATL	Achilles tendon	COMP	
	lengthening	AUGIB	acute upper gastrointesti-
	adult T-cell leukemia		nal bleeding
	anterior tricuspid leaflet	AUL	acute undifferentiated
	atypical lymphocytes		leukemia
ATLL	adult T-cell leukemia	AUR	acute urinary retention
	lymphoma	AUS	acute urethral syndrome
ATLS	advanced trauma life		auscultation
	support	AUTO SP	automatic speech
ATM	acute transverse myelitis	AV	anteverted
	atmosphere		arteriovenous
At ma	atrial milliamp		atrioventricular
ATN	acute tubular necrosis		auditory visual
ATNC	atraumatic normocephalic		auriculoventricular
aTNM	autopsy staging of cancer	AVA	aortic valve atresia
ATNR	asymmetrical tonic neck		arteriovenous anastomosis
	reflex	AVB	atrioventricular block
ATP	addiction treatment	AVC	acrylic veneer crown
	program	AVD	aortic valve disease
	adenosine triphosphate		apparent volume of
	anterior tonsillar pillar		distribution
	autoimmune	AVDP	asparaginase, vincristine,
	thrombocytopenia		daunorubicin, and
	purpura		prednisone
ATPase	adenosine triphosphatase		avoirdupois
ATPS	ambient temperature &	AVDO2	arteriovenous oxygen
	pressure, saturated with		difference
	water vapor	AVF	arteriovenous fistula

	augmented unipolar foot (left leg)	AWOL	absent without leave
avg	average	AWU	alcohol withdrawal unit
AVGs	ambulatory visit groups	ax	axillary
AVH	acute viral hepatitis	AXB	axillary block
AVJR	atrioventricular junctional rhythm	AXC	aortic cross clamp
AVL	augmented unipolar left (left arm)	ax-fem.fem.	axilla-femoral-femoral (graft)
AVM	atriovenous malformation	AXR	abdomen x-ray
AVN	arteriovenous nicking	AXT	alternating exotropia
	atrioventricular node	AZA	azathioprine (Imuran®)
	avascular necrosis	AZA-CR	azacitidine
AVNRT	atrioventricular node recovery time	5-AZC	azacitidine
	atrioventricular nodal reentry tachycardia	AzdU	azidouridine
		AZQ	diaziquone
A-VO$_2$	arteriovenous oxygen difference	AZT	zidovudine (azidothymidine)
AVOC	avocation	A-Z test	Aschheim-Zondek test (diagnostic test for pregnancy)
AVP	arginine vasopressin		
AVR	aortic valve replacement augmented unipolar right (right arm)		

B

AVRT	atrioventricular reciprocating tachycardia		
AVS	atriovenous shunt		
AVSS	afebrile, vital signs stable	B	bacillus
AVT	atrioventricular tachycardia		bands
	atypical ventricular tachycardia		bilateral
			black
			bloody
AW	abdominal wall		both
	abnormal wave		brother
	airway		botulism (Vaccine B is botulism toxoid)
A/W	able to work		
A&W	alive and well		buccal
AWA	alcohol withdrawal assessment	B$_1$	thiamine HCl
		BI & II	Billroth I and II
	as well as	B$_2$	riboflavin
A waves	atrial contraction wave	B$_3$	nicotinic acid
AWB	autologous whole blood	b/4	before
AWDW	assault with a deadly weapon	B$_5$	pantothenic acid
		-B$_6$	pyridoxine HCl
AWI	anterior wall infarct	B$_7$	biotin
AWMI	anterior wall myocardial infarction	B$_8$	adenosine phosphate
		B$_{12}$	cyanocobalamin
AWO	airway obstruction	Ba	barium

21

BA	backache	BANS	back, arm, neck and scalp
	Baptist	BAO	basal acid output
	benzyl alcohol	BAP	blood agar plate
	bile acid	Barb	barbiturate
	blood alcohol	BARN	bilateral acute retinal
	bone age		necrosis
	Bourns assist	BAS	boric acid solution
	branchial artery	BaS	barium swallow
	broken appointment	BASK	basket cells
	bronchial asthma	baso.	basophil
B > A	bone greater than air	BASO	basophilic stippling
B & A	brisk and active	STIP	
Bab	Babinski	BAT	Behavioral Avoidance
BAC	benzalkonium chloride		Test
	blood alcohol		brightness acuity tester
	concentration	BATO	boronic acid adduct of
	buccoaxiocervical		technetium dioxime
BACI	bovine anti-	batt	battery
	cryptosporidium	BAVP	balloon aortic
	immunoglobulin		valvuloplasty
BACON	bleomycin, doxorubicin,	BAW	bronchoalveolar washing
	lomustine, vincristine,	BB	baby boy
	and mechlorethamine		backboard
BACOP	bleomycin, Adriamycin®,		bad breath
	cyclophosphamide,		bed bath
	vincristine, and		bed board
	prednisone		beta-blocker
BACT	bacteria		blanket bath
	base activated clotting		blood bank
	time		blow bottle
BAD	dipolar affective disorder		blue bloaters
BaE	barium enema		body belts
BAE	bronchial artery		both bones
	embolization		breakthrough bleeding
BAEP	brain stem auditory		breast biopsy
	evoked potential		brush biopsy
BAERs	brain stem auditory		buffer base
	evoked responses	B&B	bowel and bladder
BAL	balance	B/B	backward bending
	blood alcohol level	BBA	born before arrival
	British antilewisite	BBB	baseball bat beating
	(dimercaprol)		blood-brain barrier
	bronchoalveolar lavage		bundle branch block
BALB	binaural alternate	BBBB	bilateral bundle branch
	loudness balance		block
BALF	bronchoalveolar lavage	BBD	before bronchodilator
	fluid		benign breast disease
BaM	barium meal	BBM	banked breast milk
BAND	band neutrophil (stab)	BBOW	bulging bag of water

22

BBS	bilateral breath sounds	BCOC	bowel care of choice
BBT	basal body temperature		bowel cathartic of choice
BB to MM	belly button to medial malleolus	BCP	birth control pills
			blood cell profile
B Bx	breast biopsy		carmustine, cyclophosphamide, and prednisone
BC	back care		
	bed and chair		
	bicycle	BCPAP	Broun's continuous positive airway pressure
	birth control		
	blood culture		
	Blue Cross	BCRS	Brief Cognitive Rate Scale
	bone conduction		
	Bourn control	BCS	battered child syndrome
B/C	because		Budd-Chiari syndrome
	blood urea nitrogen/ creatinine ratio	BCU	burn care unit
		BD	band neutrophil
B&C	bed and chair		base down
	biopsy and curettage		bile duct
	board and care		birth date
	breathed and cried		birth defect
BCBR	bilateral carotid body resection		blood donor
			brain dead
BC/BS	Blue Cross/Blue Shield		bronchial drainage
BCA	balloon catheter angioplasty	BDAE	Boston Diagnostic Aphasia Examination
	basal cell atypia	BDBS	Bonnet-Dechaume-Blanc syndrome
	brachiocephalic artery		
BCAA	branched-chain amino acids	BDC	burn-dressing change
		BDE	bile duct exploration
B. cat	*Branhamella catarrhalis*	BDF	black divorced female
B-CAVe	bleomycin, lomustine, doxorubicin, and vinblastine	BDI	Beck Depression Inventory
		BDI SF	Beck's Depression Inventory-Short Form
BCC	basal cell carcinoma		
	birth control clinic	BDL	below detectable limits
BCCa	basal cell carcinoma		bile duct ligation
BCD	basal cell dysplasia	BDM	black divorced male
BCE	basal cell epithelioma	B-DOPA	bleomycin, dacarbazine, vincristine, prednisone, and doxorubicin
B cell	large lymphocyte		
BCG	bacille Calmette-Guérin vaccine		
		BDP	beclomethasone dipropionate
	bicolor guaiac		
BCL	basic cycle length		best demonstrated practice
BCM	below costal margin	BDR	background diabetic retinopathy
	birth control medication		
	body cell mass	BE	bacterial endocarditis
BCNP	Board Certified Nuclear Pharmacist		barium enema
			base excess
BCNU	carmustine		below elbow

23

	bread equivalent	BGC	basal-ganglion calcification
	breast examination		
B↑E	both upper extremities	BGCT	benign glandular cell tumor
B↓E	both lower extremities		
B & E	brisk and equal	BGDC	Bartholin gland duct cyst
BEA	below elbow amputation	BGL	blood glucose level
BEAM	brain electrical activity mapping	BGM	blood glucose monitoring
		BH	breath holding
BEC	bacterial endocarditis	BHC	benzene hexachloride
BED	biochemical evidence of disease	BHD	carmustine, hydroxyurea, and dacarbazine
BEE	basal energy expenditure	B-HEXOS-A-LK	beta hexosaminidase A leukocytes
BEF	bronchoesophageal fistula		
BEH	benign essential hypertension	BHI	biosynthetic human insulin
Beh Sp	behavior specialist	BHN	bridging hepatic necrosis
BEI	butanol-extractable iodine	BHR	bronchial hyperrespon-siveness
BEP	bleomycin, etoposide, and cisplatin		
		BHP	boarding home placement
	brain stem evoked potentials	BHS	beta-hemolytic streptococci
			breath-holding spell
BEV	billion electron volts	BHT	breath hydrogen test
	bleeding esophageal varices	BI	base in
			brain injury
BF	black female		bowel impaction
	boyfriend	Bi	bismuth
	breakfast fed	BIB	brought in by
	breast-feed	BIC	brain injury center
B/F	bound-to-free ratio	Bicarb	bicarbonate
BFA	baby for adoption	BiCNU®	carmustine
	bifemoral arteriogram	BICROS	bilateral contralateral routing of signals
BFC	benign febrile convulsion		
bFGF	basic fibroblast growth factor	BICU	burn intensive care unit
		BID	brought in dead
BFL	breast firm and lactating		twice daily
BFM	black married female	BIDA	amonafide
BFP	biologic false positive	BIDS	bedtime insulin, daytime sulfonylurea
B. frag	Bacillus fragilis		
BFT	bentonite flocculation test	BIF	bifocal
	biofeedback training	BIG	botulism immune globulin
BFU_e	erythroid burst-forming unit	BIG 6	analysis of 6 serum components (see SMA 6)
BG	baby girl		
	blood glucose	BIH	benign intracranial hypertension
	bone graft		
B-G	Bender Gestalt (test)		bilateral inguinal hernia
B-GA-LACTO	beta galactosidase	BIL	bilateral
			brother-in-law

BILAT SLC	bilateral short leg case		BLBK	blood bank
			BLBS	bilateral breath sounds
BILAT SXO	bilateral salpingo-oophorectomy		BL = BS	bilateral equal breath sounds
Bili	bilirubin		bl cult	blood culture
BILI-C	conjugated bilirubin		B-L-D	breakfast, lunch, and dinner
BIL MRY	bilateral myringotomy			
BIMA	bilateral internal mammary arteries		bldg	bleeding
			bld tm	bleeding time
BIN	twice a night (this is a dangerous abbreviation)		BLE	both lower extremities
			BLEO	bleomycin sulfate
BIOF	biofeedback		BLESS	bath, laxative, enema, shampoo, and shower
BIP	bipolar affective disorder			
BiPD	biparietal diameter		BLL	bilateral lower lobe
bisp	bispinous diameter		BLM	bleomycin sulfate
B.I.W.	twice a week (this is a dangerous abbreviation)		BLOBS	bladder obstruction
			BLPO	beta-lactamase-producing organism
BIZ-PLT	bizarre platelets			
BJ	Bence Jones		BLQ	both lower quadrants
	biceps jerk		BLR	blood flow rate
	body jacket		BLS	basic life support
	bone and joint		B.L. unit	Bessey-Lowry units
BJE	bones, joints, and extremities		BM	black male
				bone marrow
BJI	bone and joint infection			bowel movement
BJM	bones, joints, and muscles			breast milk
			BMA	biomedical application
BJP	Bence Jones protein			bone marrow aspirate
BK	below knee (amputation)		BMC	bone marrow cells
	bradykinin		BMD	Becker muscular dystrophy
	bullous keratopathy			
BKA	below knee amputation			bone marrow depression
BKC	blepharokerato-conjunctivitis			bone mineral density
			BME	biomedical engineering
bkft	breakfast			brief maximal effort
Bkg	background		BMI	body mass index
BKU	base up		BMJ	bones, muscles, joints
BKWP	below-knee walking plaster (cast)		BMK	birthmark
			BMM	black married male
BL	baseline (fetal heart rate)		BMP	behavior management plan
	bland		BMR	basal metabolic rate
	blast cells			best motor response
	blood level		BMT	bilateral myringotomy and tubes
	blood loss			
	bronchial lavage			bone marrow transplant
	Burkitt's lymphoma		BMTN	bone marrow transplant neutropenia
BLB	Boothby-Lovelace-Bulbulian (oxygen mask)			
			BMTT	bilateral myringotomy with tympanic tubes

BMTU	bone marrow transplant unit		British Pharmacopeia
BMU	basic multicellular unit		bullous pemphigoid
BN	bladder neck		bypass
BNC	binasal cannula	BP-200	Bourn's Infant Pressure Ventilator
	bladder neck contracture	BPI	bipolar affective disorder, Type I
BNCT	boron neutron capture therapy	BPD	biparietal diameter
BNI	blind nasal intubation		borderline personality disorder
BNL	below normal limits		
	breast needle localization		bronchopulmonary dysplasia
BNO	bladder neck obstruction		
BNR	bladder neck retraction	BPd	diastolic blood pressure
BNS	benign nephrosclerosis	BPF	bronchopleural fistula
BO	base out	BPH	benign prostatic hypertrophy
	behavior objective		
	body odor	BPG	bypass graft
	bowel obstruction	BPI	bactericidal/permeability increasing (protein)
B & O	belladonna & opium (suppositories)	BPL	benzylpenicilloylpoly-lysine
BOA	born on arrival		
	born out of asepsis	BPLA	blood pressure, left arm
BOB	ball on back	BPM	beats per minute
BOD	bilateral orbital decompression		breaths per minute
		BPN	bacitracin, polymyxin B, and neomycin sulfate
Bod Units	Bodansky units		
BOE	bilateral otitis externa	BPO	bilateral partial oophorectomy
BOLD	bleomycin, vincristine (Oncovin®), lomustine, and dacarbazine		
		BPP	biophysical profile
		BPPP	bilateral pedal pulses present
BOM	bilateral otitis media		
BOMA	bilateral otitis media, acute	BPPV	benign paroxysmal postural vertigo
BOO	bladder outlet obstruction	BPR	blood per rectum
BOOP	bronchitis obliterans with organized pneumonia		blood pressure recorder
		BPRS	Brief Psychiatric Rating Scale
BOT	base of tongue		
BOVR	Bureau of Vocational Rehabilitation	BPS	bilateral partial salpingectomy
		BPs	systolic blood pressure
BOW	bag of water	BPSD	bronchopulmonary segmental drainage
BOW-I	bag of water-intact		
BOW-R	bag of water-ruptured	BPV	benign paroxysmal vertigo
BP	bathroom privileges		
	bed pan		bovine papilloma virus
	bench press	Bq	becquerel
	benzoyl peroxide	BR	bathroom
	bipolar		bedrest
	birthplace		Benzing retrograde
	blood pressure		

26

	birthing room	B & S	Bartholin and Skene
	blink reflex		(glands)
	bowel rest	BSA	body surface area
	bridge		bowel sounds active
	brown	BSAB	Balthazar Scales of
Br	bromide		Adaptive Behavior
	bromine	BSB	bedside bag
BRA	brain		body surface burned
BRADY	bradycardia	BSC	bedside care
BRAO	branch retinal artery		bedside commode
	occlusion		burn scar contracture
BRAT	bananas, rice cereal,	BSCC	bedside commode chair
	applesauce, and toast	BSD	baby soft diet
BRATT	bananas, rice, cereal,		bedside drainage
	applesauce, tea, &	BSE	bovine spongiform
	toast		encephalopathy
BRB	blood-retinal barrier		breast self-examination
	bright red blood	BSEC	bedside easy chair
BRBR	bright red blood per	BSepF	black separated female
	rectum	BSepM	black separated male
BRBPR	bright red blood per	BSER	brain stem evoked
	rectum		responses
BRCM	below right costal margin	BSF	black single female
BRex	breathing exercise		busulfan
Br. Fdg.	breast-feeding	BSG	Bagolini striated glasses
BRJ	brachial radialis jerk	BSGA	beta streptococcus group A
BRM	biological response	BSI	body substance isolation
	modifiers		brain stem injury
BRO	brother	BSL	blood sugar level
BRONK	bronchoscopy	BS L	breath sounds diminished,
BRP	bathroom privileges	base	left base
BR RAO	branch retinal artery	BSM	black single male
	occlusion	BSN	Bachelor of Science in
BR RVO	branch retinal vein		Nursing
	occlusion		bowel sounds normal
Br.S.	breath sounds	BSNA	bowel sounds normal and
BRU	basic remodeling unit		active
	(osteon)	BSNMT	Bachelor of Science in
BRVO	branch retinal vein		Nuclear Medicine
	occlusion		Technology
BS	barium swallow	BSNT	breast soft and nontender
	bedside	BSO	bilateral salpingo-
	before sleep		oophorectomy
	Bennett seal		l-buthionine sulfoximine
	blood sugar	BSOM	bilateral serous otitis
	Blue Shield		media
	bowel sounds	BSP	Bromsulphalein®
	breath sounds	BSPA	bowel sounds present and
			active

BSPM	body surface potential mapping	BTL	bilateral tubal ligation
		BTO	bilateral tubal occlusion
BSRT (R)	Bachelor of Science in Radiologic Technology (Registered)	BTPABA	bentiromide
		BTPS	body temperature pressure saturated
BSS	bedside scale	BTR	bladder tumor recheck
	bismuth subsalicylate	BU	base up (prism)
	black silk sutures		below umbilicus
BSS®	balanced salt solution		Bodansky units
BSSG	sitogluside		burn unit
BSSO	bilateral sagittal split osteotomy	BUdR	bromodeoxyuridine
		BUE	both upper extremities
BSSS	benign sporadic sleep spikes	BUFA	baby up for adoption
		BUN	blood urea nitrogen
BST	bedside testing	BUR	back-up rate (ventilator)
	bovine somatotropin	Burd	Burdick suction
	brief stimulus therapy	BUS	Bartholin, urethral, and Skene's glands
BSU	Bartholin, Skene's, urethra (glands)		
		BV	bacterial vaginitis
	Base Service Unit		biological value
BSW	Bachelor of Social Work		blood volume
BT	bedtime	BVAD	biventricular assist device
	behavioral therapy	BVE	blood volume expander
	bituberous	BVL	bilateral vas ligation
	bladder tumor	BVM	bag valve mask
	Blalock-Taussig (shunt)	BVO	branch vein occlusion
	bleeding time	BVR	Bureau of Vocational Rehabilitation
	blood type		
	blood transfusion	BVRT	Benton Visual Retention Test
	brain tumor		
	breast tumor	BVT	bilateral ventilation tubes
BTA	below the ankle	BW	birth weight
BTB	back to bed		bite-wing (radiograph)
	beat-to-beat (variability)		body water
	break-through bleeding		body weight
BTBV	beat to beat variability	B & W	Black and White (milk of magnesia & aromatic cascara fluidextract)
BTC	bladder tumor check		
	by the clock		
BTE	Baltimore Therapeutic Equipment (work simulator)	BWA	bed wetter admission
		BWCS	bagged white cell study
	behind-the-ear (hearing aid)	BWFI	bacteriostatic water for injection
BTF	blenderized tube feeding	BWidF	black widowed female
BTFS	breast tumor frozen section	BWidM	black widowed male
		BWS	battered woman syndrome
BTG	beta thromboglobulin	BWs	bite-wing (x-rays)
BTI	biliary tract infection	BWX	bite-wing x-ray
	bitubal interruption	Bx	biopsy

BX BS	Blue Cross and Blue Shield
BXM	B cell crossmatch
ΦBZ	phenylbutazone
BZD	benzodiazepine
BZDZ	benzodiazepine

C

C	ascorbic acid
	carbohydrate
	Catholic
	Caucasian
	Celsius
	centigrade
	clubbing
	constricted
	cyanosis
	hundred
c̄	with
$C_1...C_7$	cervical nerve 1 through 7
	cervical vertebra 1 through 7
C_1 to C_9	precursor molecules of the complement system
C3	complement C3
C4	complement C4
CII	controlled substance, class 2
C_{II}	second cranial nerve
CA	cancelled appointment
	carcinoma
	cardiac arrest
	carotid artery
	celiac artery
	chronologic age
	Cocaine Anonymous
	compressed air
	continuous aerosol
	coronary angioplasty
	coronary artery
Ca	calcium
CA 125	cancer antigen 125

C&A	Clinitest® and Acetest®
CAA	crystalline amino acids
CAB	catheter-associated bacteriuria
	cellulose acetate butyrate
	coronary artery bypass
CABG	coronary artery bypass graft
CaBI	calcium bone index
CABS	coronary artery bypass surgery
CAC	cardioacceleratory center
	Certified Alcohol Counselor
	Community Action Center
CACI	computer-assisted continuous infusion
$CaCO_3$	calcium carbonate
CACP	cisplatin
CAD	coronary artery disease
CADD®	Computerized Ambulatory Drug Delivery (pump)
CADP	computer-assisted design of prosthesis
CAE	cellulose acetate electrophoresis
	cyclophosphamide, doxorubicin, and etoposide
CAEC	cardiac arrhythmia evaluation center
CaEDTA	calcium disodium edetate
CAF	chronic atrial fibrillation
	cyclophosphamide, doxorubicin, and fluorouracil
CAFT	Clinitron® air fluidized therapy
CAG	chronic atrophic gastritis
	continuous ambulatory gamma globin (infusion)
CaG	calcium gluconate
CAGE	a questionnaire for alcoholism evaluation (JAMA 1984; 252: 1905-7)
CAH	chronic active hepatitis
	chronic aggressive hepatitis

	congenital adrenal hyperplasia		compound action potentials
CAI	carbonic anhydrase inhibitors		cyclophosphamide, doxorubicin, and cisplatin
	carboxyamide aminoimidazoles	CaP	carcinoma of the prostate
CAIV	cold-adapted influenza virus vaccine	Ca/P	calcium to phosphorus ratio
CAL	callus	CAPB	central auditory processing battery
	calories (cal)		
	chronic airflow limitation	CAPD	chronic ambulatory peritoneal dialysis
cal ct	calorie count		
CALD	chronic active liver disease	CAR	cardiac ambulation routine
CALGB	Cancer and Leukemia Group B	CARB	carbohydrate
		CARBO	Carbocaine®
CALLA	common acute lymphoblastic leukemia antigen	CARD	Cardiac Automatic Resuscitative Device
CAM	Caucasian adult male	CARN	Certified Addiction Registered Nurse
	child abuse management	CAS	carotid artery stenosis
	confusion assessment method		Chemical Abstract Service
CAMD	computer-aided molecular design		Clinical Asthma Score
CAMF	cyclophosphamide, adriamycin, methotrexate, and fluorouracil	CASA	computer-assisted semen analysis
		CASHD	coronary arteriosclerotic heart disease
CAMP	cyclophosphamide, doxorubicin, methotrexate, and procarbazine	CASP	Child Analytic Study Program
		CASS	computer-aided sleep system
cAMP	cyclic adenosine monophosphate	CAST®	color allergy screening test
CAN	contrast-associated nephropathy	CAT	carnitine acetyl transferase
			cataract
	cord around neck		Children's Apperception Test
CA/N	child abuse and neglect		
CANC	cancelled		computed axial tomography
CANP	Certified Adult Nurse Practitioner	CATH	catheter
			catheterization
CAO	chronic airway (airflow) obstruction		Catholic
		CATS	catecholamines
CAP	capsule	CAU	Caucasian
	chloramphenicol	CAV	computer-aided ventilation
	community-acquired pneumonia		

	cyclophosphamide, doxorubicin, and vincristine	
CAVB	complete atrioventricular block	
CAVC	common artrioventricular canal	
CAVH	continuous atriovenous hemofiltration	
CAVHD	continuous arteriovenous hemodialysis	
CAV-P-VP	cyclophosphamide, doxorubicin, vincristine, cisplatin, and etoposide	
CAVU	continuous arteriovenous ultrafiltration	
CB	cesarean birth chronic bronchitis code blue	
C & B	chair and bed crown and bridge	
CBA	chronic bronchitis and asthma	
CBC	carbenicillin complete blood count	
CBCDA	carboplatin	
CBCT	community based clinical trials	
CBD	closed bladder drainage common bile duct	
CBDE	common bile duct exploration	
CBER	Center for Biologics Evaluation and Research	
CBF	cerebral blood flow	
CBFS	cerebral blood flow studies	
CBFV	cerebral blood flow velocity	
CBG	capillary blood glucose	
CBI	continuous bladder irrigation	
CBN	chronic benign neutropenia collected by nurse	
CBP	chronic benign pain copper-binding protein	

CBPS	coronary bypass surgery
CBR	carotid bodies resected chronic bedrest complete bedrest
CBRAM	controlled partial rebreathing-anesthesia method
CBS	chronic brain syndrome coarse breath sounds Cruveilhier-Baumgarten syndrome
CBZ	carbamazepine
CC	cardiac catheterization Catholic cerebral concussion chief complaint chronic complainer circulatory collapse clean catch (urine) coracoclavicular cord compression corpus collosum creatinine clearance critical condition cubic centimeter (cc), (mL) with correction (with glasses)
C_c	concentration of drug in the central compartment
C/C	cholecystectomy and operative cholangio-gram complete upper and lower dentures
CCII	Clinical Clerk–2nd year
C & C	cold and clammy
CCA	circumflex coronary artery common carotid artery concentrated care area
CCAP	capsule cartilage articular preservation
CCB	calcium channel blocker(s)
CCC	Cancer Care Center child care clinic Comprehensive Cancer Center

CC & C	colony count and culture
CCC-A	Certificate of Clinical Competence in Audiology
CCC-SP	Certificate of Clinical Competence in Speech-Language Pathology
CCD	change-coupled device
	childhood celiac disease
CCE	clubbing, cyanosis, and edema
	countercurrent electrophoresis
CCF	compound comminuted fracture
	crystal-induced chemotactic factor
CCFE	cyclophosphamide, cisplatin, fluorouracil, and estramustine
CCHD	cyanotic congenital heart disease
CCI	chronic coronary insufficiency
CCK	cholecystokinin
CCK-OP	cholecystokinin octapeptide
CCK-PZ	cholecystokinin pancreozymin
CCL	cardiac catheterization laboratory
	critical condition list
CCl$_4$	carbon tetrachloride
CCM	calcium citrate malate
	cyclophosphamide, lomustine, and methotrexate
CCMSU	clean catch midstream urine
CCMU	critical care medicine unit
CCN	continuing care nursery
CCNS	cell cycle-nonspecific
CCNU	lomustine
C-collar	cervical collar
CCPD	continuous cycling (cyclical) peritoneal dialysis
CCR	cardiac care reversal

	cardiac catheterization recovery
	continuous complete remission
	counterclockwise rotation
C$_{cr}$	creatinine clearance
CCRC	continuing care residential community
CCRN	Certified Critical Care Registered Nurse
CCRU	critical care recovery unit
CCS	cell cycle-specific
CCT	calcitriol
	Certified Cardiographic Technician
	closed cerebral trauma
	closed cranial trauma
	congenitally corrected transposition (of the great vessels)
	crude coal tar
CCTGA	congenitally corrected transposition of the great arteries
CCT in PET	crude coal tar in petroleum
CCTV	closed circuit television
CCU	coronary care unit
	critical care unit
CCUA	clean catch urinalysis
CCUP	colpocystourethropexy
CCV	Critical Care Ventilator (Ohio)
CCW	childcare worker
	counterclockwise
CCX	complications
CCY	cholecystectomy
CD	cadaver donor
	candela
	cervical dystonia
	cesarean delivery
	character disorder
	chemical dependency
	childhood disease
	chronic dialysis
	common duct
	communication disorders
	complicated delivery
	conjugate diameter

	continuous drainage		congenital diaphragmatic
	convulsive disorder		hernia
	Crohn's disease		congenital dislocation of
	cyclodextran		hip
	cytarabine and		congenital dysplasia of
	daunorubicin		the hip
Cd	cadmium	CDI	Children's Depression
	concentration of drug		Inventory
C/D	cigarettes per day		Cotrel Duobosset
	cup to disc ratio		Instrumentation
CD4	helper-inducer T-cell	C Dif	*Clostridium difficile*
CD8	suppressor-cytotoxic	CDK	climatic droplet
	T-cell		keratopathy
C&D	curettage and desiccation	CDLE	chronic discoid lupus
	cystectomy and diversion		erythematosus
	cytoscopy and dilatation	CDP	Child Development
CDA	Certified Dental Assistant		Program
	chenodeoxycholic acid	CDQ	corrected development
	(chenodiol)		quotient
	congenital dyserythropoie-	CDR	Clinical Dementia Rating
	tic anemia		continuing disability
2CdA	chlorodeoxyadenosine		review
CDAI	Crohn's Disease Activity	CDR(H)	cup-to-disc ratio
	Index		horizontal
CDAK	Cordis Dow Artificial	CDR(V)	cup-to-disc ratio vertical
	Kidney	CDU	chemical dependency unit
CDAP	continuous distended	CDV	canine distemper virus
	airway pressure	CDX	chlordiazepoxide
CDB	cough and deep breath	cdyn	dynamic compliance
CDC	calculated day of	CE	California encephalitis
	confinement		capillary electrophoresis
	cancer detection center		cardiac enlargement
	carboplatin, doxorubicin,		cardioesophageal
	and cyclophosphamide		cataract extraction
	Centers for Disease		central episiotomy
	Control		community education
	Certified Drug Counselor		continuing education
	chenodeoxycholic acid		contrast echocardiology
CDCA	chenodeoxycholic acid	C&E	consultation and
	(chenodiol)		examination
CDD	Certificate of Disability		cough and exercise
	for Discharge		curettage and
CDDP	cisplatin		electrodesiccation
CDE	canine distemper	CEA	carcinoembryonic antigen
	encephalitis		carotid endarterectomy
	Certified Diabetes	CEC	Council for Exceptional
	Educator		Children
	common duct exploration	CECT	contrast enhancement
CDH	chronic daily headache		computed tomography

CEI	continuous extravascular infusion		complete Freund's adjuvant
CEL	cardiac exercise laboratory	CFAC	complement-fixing antibody consumption
CEN	Certified (Nurse)–Emergency Room	C-factor	cleverness factor
CEO	chief executive officer	CFF	critical fusion (flicker) frequency
CEP	cardiac enzyme panel	CFI	confrontation fields intact
	cognitive evoked potential	CFIDS	chronic fatigue immune dysfunction syndrome
	congenital erythropoietic porphyria	CFL	cisplatin, fluorouracil, and leucovorin calcium
	countercurrent electrophoresis	CFLX	ciprofloxacin
CEPH	cephalic	CFM	close fitting mask
	cephalosporin		craniofacial microsomia
CEPH FLOC	cephalin flocculation		cyclophosphamide, fluorouracil, and citoxantrone
CER	conditioned emotional response	CFNS	chills, fever, and night sweats
CE&R	central episiotomy and repair	CFP	cystic fibrosis protein
CERA	cortical evoked response audiometry	CFPT	cyclophosphamide, fluorouracil, prednisone, and tamoxifen
CERD	chronic end-stage renal disease	CFS	cancer family syndrome
CERULO	ceruloplasmin		Child and Family Service
CERV	cervical		chronic fatigue syndrome
CES	cognitive environmental stimulation	CFT	complement fixation test
	estrogen, conjugated (conjugated estrogen substance)	CF test	complement fixation test
		CFU	colony-forming units
CEV	cyclophosphamide, etoposide, and vincristine	CFU-E	colony-forming unit–erythroid
		CFU-G	colony-forming unit–granulocyte
CF	calcium leucovorin (citrovorum factor)	CFU-G/M	colony-forming unit–granulocyte/macro-phage
	cancer-free		
	cardiac failure	CFU-M	colony-forming unit–macrophage
	Caucasian female		
	Christmas factor	CFU-S	colony-forming unit–spleen
	cisplatin and fluorouracil		
	complement fixation	CG	cardiogreen (dye)
	contractile force		cholecystogram
	count fingers		contact guarding
	cystic fibrosis	CGB	chronic gastrointestinal (tract) bleeding
C&F	cell and flare		
	chills and fever	CGD	chronic granulomatous disease
CFA	common femoral artery		

CGI	Clinical Global Impressions (scale)		doxorubicin, and cisplatin
CGL	chronic granulocytic leukemia	CHARGE	Columbus (of eyes), hearing deficit, choanal
	with correction/with glasses		atresia, retardation of growth, genital defects
CGN	chronic glomerulonephri-tis		(males only), and endocardial cushion
CGS	catgut suture		defect
CGTT	cortisol glucose tolerance test	CHB	complete heart block
cGy	centigray	CHBHA	congenital Heinz body hemolytic anemia
CH	chest	CH_{3-} CCNU	semustine
	chief		
	child (children)	cHct	central hematocrit
	chronic	CHD	center hemodialysis
	cluster headache		childhood diseases
	congenital hypothyroidism		chronic hemodialysis
	convalescent hospital		common hepatic duct
	crown-heal		congenital heart disease
CHL	conductive hearing loss		coordinate home care
CHN	central hemorrhagic necrosis	CHEM 7	laboratory tests for glucose, blood urine
c̄ hold	withhold		nitrogen, creatinine,
ch¹	Christ Church chromosone		potassium, sodium, chloride, and carbon
CH50	total hemolytic complement		dioxide
CHA	compound hypermetropic astigmatism	CHEMO	chemotherapy
		ChemoRx	chemotherapy
		CHESS	chemical shift selective
CHAD	cyclophosphamide, Adriamycin®, cisplatin,	CHF	congestive heart failure Crimean hemorrhagic
	and hexamethyl-melamine		fever
CHAI	continuous hepatic artery infusion	CHFV	combined high frequency of ventilation
CHAM-OCA	cyclophosphamide, hydroxyurea,	CHG	change
		CHI	closed head injury
	dactinomycin, methotrexate,		creatinine-height index
		CHIP	iproplatin
	vincristine, leucovorin,	Chix	chickenpox
	and doxorubicin	CHN	community nursing home
CHAM-PUS	Civilian Health and Medical Program of the	CHO	carbohydrate
		chol	cholesterol
	Uniformed Services	CHOP	cyclophosphamide,
CHAP	child health associate practitioner		doxorubicin, vincristine, prednisone
	cyclophosphamide, hexamethylmelamine,	CHPX	chickenpox
		CHR	Cercaria-Hullen reaction chronic

CHRS	congenital hereditary retinoschisis		polyradiculoneuropathy
CHS	Chediak-Higashi syndrome	CIDS	cellular immunodeficiency syndrome
CHT	closed head trauma		continuous insulin delivery system
CHU	closed head unit	CIE	chemotherapy induced emesis
CHUC	Certified Health Unit Coordinator		counterimmunoelectro-phoresis
CI	cardiac index		crossed immunoelectro-phoresis
	cesium implant		
	Clinical Instructor	CIEA	continuous infusion epidural analgesia
	cochlear implant		
	complete iridectomy	CIEP	counterimmunoelectro-phoresis
	continuous infusion		
	coronary insufficiency	CIG	cigarettes
Ci	curie(s)	CIHD	chronic ischemic heart disease
CIA	calcaneal insufficiency avulsion	CII	continuous insulin infusion
	chronic idiopathic anhidrosis	CIIA	common internal iliac artery
CIAA	competitive insulin autoantibodies	CIN	cervical intraepithelial neoplasia
CIAED	collagen induced autoimmune ear disease		chemotherapy induced neutropenia
CIB	Carnation Instant Breakfast®		chronic interstitial nephritis
	crying-induced bronchospasm	CINE	chemotherapy-induced nausea and emesis
	cytomegalic inclusion bodies		cineangiogram
CIBD	chronic inflammatory bowel disease	CIP	Cardiac Injury Panel
CIBP	chronic intractable benign pain	CIPD	chronic intermittent peritoneal dialysis
CIC	cardioinhibitory center	Circ	circulation
	circulating immune complexes		circumcision
			circumference
	clean intermittent catheterization	circ. & sen.	circulation and sensation
	coronary intensive care	CIS	carcinoma in situ
CICE	combined intracapsular cataract extraction	CI&S	conjunctival irritation and swelling
CICU	cardiac intensive care unit	CISCA	cisplatin, cyclophospha-mide, and doxorubicin
CID	cervical immobilization device	Cis-DDP	cisplatin
	cytomegalic inclusion disease	CIT	conventional immunosuppressive therapy
CIDP	chronic inflammatory demyelinating		

	conventional insulin therapy	CLLE	columnar-lined lower esophagus
CITP	capillary isotachophoresis	cl liq	clear liquid
CIU	chronic idiopathic urticaria	Cl_{nr}	nonrenal clearance
CJD	Creutzfeldt-Jakob disease	CLO	Campylobacter-like organism
CJR	centric jaw relation		close
CK	check		cod liver oil
	creatine kinase	CL & P	cleft lip and palate
CK-BB	creatine kinase BB band	Cl_r	renal clearance
CKC	cold knife conization	CLRO	community leave for reorientation
CK-ISO	creatine kinase isoenzyme	CLS	capillary leak syndrome
CK-MB	creatine kinase MB band	CLSE	calf lung surfactant extract (Infasurf®)
CK MM	creatine kinase MM band	CLT	chronic lymphocytic thyroiditis
CKW	clockwise		cool lace tent
Cl	chloride	Cl_T	total body clearance
CL	clear liquid	CL VOID	clean voided specimen
	cleft lip	clysis	hypodermoclysis
	cloudy	cm	centimeter
	critical list	CM	capreomycin
	cycle length		cardiac monitor
	lung compliance		Caucasian male
C_L	compliance of the lungs		centimeter (cm)
CLA	community living arrangements		chondromalacia
CLASS	computer laser assisted surgical system		cochlear microphonics
			common migraine
Clav	clavicle		continuous murmur
CLB	chlorambucil		contrast media
CLBBB	complete left bundle branch block		costal margin
CLC	cork leather and celastic (orthotic)		cow's milk
			culture media
CL/CP	cleft lip and cleft palate		cystic mesothelioma
CLD	chronic liver disease		tomorrow morning (this is a dangerous abbreviation)
	chronic lung disease		
Cl_d	dialysis clearance		
CLE	centrilobular emphysema		
	continuous lumbar epidural (anesthetic)	cm^3	cubic centimeter
CLF	cholesterol-lecithin flocculation	CMA	compound myopic astigmatism
CLG	clorgyline	CMAF	centrifuged microaggregate filter
CLH	chronic lobular hepatitis		
Cl_h	hepatic clearance	CMAPs	compound muscle action potentials
CLI	clomipramine		
Cl_{int}	intrinsic clearance	C_{max}	maximum concentration of drug
CLL	chronic lymphocytic leukemia	CMB	carbolic methylene blue

CMBBT	cervical mucous basal body temperature	CMK	congenital multicystic kidney
CMC	carpal metacarpal (joint)	CML	cell-mediated lympholysis
	carboxymethylcellulose		chronic myelogenous leukemia
	chloramphenicol	CMM	Comprehensive Major Medical (insurance)
	chronic mucocutaneous candidosis		cutaneous malignant melanoma
	closed mitral commissurotomy	CMML	chronic myelomacrocytic leukemia
CMD	cytomegalic disease		
CME	cervicomediastinal exploration (examination)	CMMS	Columbia Mental Maturity Scale
	continuing medical education	CMO	Chief Medical Officer
			consult made out
	cystoid macular edema	CMP	cardiomyopathy
CMER	current medical evidence of record		chondromalacia patellae
			cushion mouthpiece
CMF	cyclophosphamide, methotrexate and fluorouracil	CMPT	cervical mucous penetration test
		CMR	cerebral metabolic rate
CMFP	cyclophosphamide, methotrexate, fluorouracil, and prednisone	CMRNG	chromosomally mediated resistant *Neisseria gonorrhoeae*
CMFT	same as CMF with tamoxifen	$CMRO_2$	cerebral metabolic rate for oxygen
CMFVP	cyclophosphamide, methotrexate, fluorouracil, vincristine, and prednisone	CMS	children's medical services
			circulation motion sensation
		CMSUA	clean midstream urinalysis
CMG	cystometrogram	CMT	carpometatarsal (joint)
CMGN	chronic membranous glomerulonephritis		Certified Medical Transcriptionist
CMHC	community mental health center		cervical motion tenderness
CMHN	Community Mental Health Nurse		Charcot-Marie tooth (disease)
CMI	cell-mediated immunity		cutis marmorata telangiectasia
	clomipramine	CMTX	chemotherapy treatment
	Cornell Medical Index	CMV	cisplatin, methotrexate, and vinblastine
CMID	cytomegalic inclusion disease		controlled mechanical ventilation
C_{min}	minimum concentration of drug		conventional mechanical ventilation
CMIR	cell-mediated immune response		cool mist vaporizer
CMJ	carpometacarpal joint		

	cytomegalovirus		Certified Orthoptist
CMVS	culture midvoid specimen		cervical orthosis
CN	cranial nerve		court order
	tomorrow night (this is a	Co	cobalt
	dangerous abbreviation)	C/O	check out
Cn	cyanide		complained of
C/N	contrast-to-noise ratio		complaints
CN II–XII	cranial nerves 2–12		under care of
CNA	Certified Nurse Aide	CO₂	carbon dioxide
	chart not available	CO₃	carbonate
CNAG	chronic narrow angle	CoA	coarctation of the aorta
	glaucoma	COAD	chronic obstructive airway
CNC	Community Nursing		disease
	Center		chronic obstructive
CNCbl	cyanocobalamin		arterial disease
CND	canned	COAG	chronic open angle
	cannot determine		glaucoma
CNDC	chronic nonspecific	COAGSC	coagulation screen
	diarrhea of childhood	COAP	cyclophosphamide,
CNE	chronic nervous		vincristine, cytarabine,
	exhaustion		and prednisone
CNF	cyclophosphamide,	COARCT	coarctation
	mitoxantrone, and	COB	cisplatin, vincristine, and
	fluorouracil		bleomycin
CNH	central neurogenic	COBS	chronic organic brain
	hypernea		syndrome
CNHC	chronodermatitis nodularis	COBT	chronic obstruction of
	helicis chronicus		biliary tract
CNM	certified nurse midwife	COC	combination oral
CNMT	Certified Nuclear		contraceptive
	Medicine Technologist	COCCIO	coccidioidomycosis
CNN	congenital nevocytic	COCM	congestive cardiomyopa-
	nevus		thy
CNOR	Certified Nurse,	COD	cataract, right eye
	Operating Room		cause of death
CNP	capillary nonprofusion		codeine
CNPS	cardiac nuclear probe		coefficient of oxygen
	scan		delivery
CNRN	Certified Neurosurgical		condition on discharge
	Registered Nurse	COD-MD	cerebro-oculardysplasia
CNS	central nervous system		muscular dystrophy
	Clinical Nurse Specialist	CODO	codocytes
CNSHA	congenital nonspherocytic	COE	court-ordered examination
	hemolytic anemia	COEPS	cortically originating
CNT	could not test		extrapyramidal
CO	carbon monoxide		symptoms
	cardiac output	COG	Central Oncology Group
	castor oil		cognitive function tests
	centric occlusion	COGN	cognition

COH carbohydrate
COHB carboxyhemoglobin
Coke Coca-Cola®
cocaine
COLD chronic obstructive lung disease
COLD A cold agglutin titer
Collyr eye wash
col/ml colonies per milliliter
colp colporrhaphy
COM chronic otitis media
COMF comfortable
COMLA cyclophosphamide, vincristine, methotrexate, calcium leucovorin, and cytarabine
COMP complications
compound
compress
cyclophosphamide, vincristine, methotrexate, and prednisone
COMT catechol-o-methyl transferase
CON A concanavalin A
conc. concentrated
CONG congenital
gallon
CONPA-DRI I cyclophosphamide, vincristine, doxorubicin, and melphalan
CONPA-DRI II conpadri I plus high-dose methotrexate
CONPA-DRI III conpadri I plus intensified doxorubicin
cont continuous
contusions
CON-TRAL contralateral
CONTU contusion
Conv. ex. convergence excess
COP cicatricial ocular pemphigoid
colloid osmotic pressure
cycophosphamide, vincristine, and prednisone

COP 1 copolymer 1
COPD chronic obstructive pulmonary disease
COPE chronic obstructive pulmonary emphysema
COPP cyclophosphamide, vincristine, procarbazine, and prednisone
COPT circumoval precipitin test
cor coronary
CORE cardiac or respiratory emergency
CORT Certified Operating Room Technician
COS cataract, left eye
Chief of Staff
clinically observed seizure
COT content of thought
COTA Certified Occupational Therapy Assistant
COTE comprehensive occupational therapy evaluation
COTX cast off to x-ray
COU cardiac observation unit
COWA controlled oral word association
COX Coxsackie virus
cytochrome C oxidase
CP centric position
cerebral palsy
Certified Paramedic
chest pain
chloroquine-primaquine combination tablets
chondromalacia patella
chronic pain
cleft palate
convenience package
creatine phosphokinase
cyclophosphamide and cisplatin
C_p concentration of drug plasma
C&P complete and pushing
cystoscopy and pyelography
CPA cardiopulmonary arrest
carotid photoangiography

	cerebellar pontile angle	CPI	constitutionally
	conditioned play		psychopathia inferior
	audiometry	CPID	chronic pelvic
	costophrenic angle		inflammatory disease
	cyclophosphamide	CPIP	chronic pulmonary
	cyproterone acetate		insufficiency of
CPAF	chlorpropamide-alcohol		prematurity
	flush	CPK	creatinine phosphokinase
CPAP	continuous positive		(BB, MB, MM are
	airway pressure		isoenzymes)
CPB	cardiopulmonary bypass	CPKD	childhood polycystic
	competitive protein		kidney disease
	binding	CPKMB	creatine phosphokinase of
CPBA	competitive protein--		muscle band
	binding assay	CPL	criminal procedure law
CPC	cerebral palsy clinic	CPM	central pontine
	chronic passive		myelinolysis
	congestion		chlorpheniramine maleate
	clinicopathologic		Clinical Practice Model
	conference		continue present
CPCR	cardiopulmonary-cerebral		management
	resuscitation		continuous passive motion
CPCS	clinical pharmacokinetics		counts per minute
	consulting service		cycles per minute
CPD	cephalopelvic		cyclophosphamide
	disproportion	CPmax	peak serum concentration
	chorioretinopathy and	CPMDI	computerized
	pituitary dysfunction		pharmacokinetic
	chronic peritoneal dialysis		model-driven drug
	citrate-phosphate-dextrose		infusion
CPDA-1	citrate-phosphate-dextrose-	CPmin	trough serum
	adenine		concentration
CPDD	calcium pyrophosphate	CPMM	constant passive motion
	deposition disease		machine
CPE	cardiogenic pulmonary	CPN	chronic pyelonephritis
	edema	CPP	central precocious puberty
	chronic pulmonary		cerebral perfusion
	emphysema		pressure
	clubbing, pitting, or		chronic pelvic pain
	edema	CPPB	continuous positive
	complete physical		pressure breathing
	examination	CPPD	calcium pyrophosphate
CPE-C	cyclopentenylcytosine		dihydrate
CPER	chest pain emergency		cisplatin
	room	CPPV	continuous positive
CPGN	chronic progressive		pressure ventilation
	glomerulonephritis	CPQ	Conner's Parent
CPH	chronic persistent		Questionnaire
	hepatitis	CPR	cardiopulmonary
			resuscitation

	tablet (French)
CPRAM	controlled partial rebreathing anesthesia method
CP/ROMI	chest pain, rule out myocardial infarction
CPRS-OCS	Comprehensive Psychiatric Rating Scale, Obsessive-Compulsive Subscale
CPS	cardiopulmonary support
	child protective services
	chloroquine-pyrimethamine sulfadoxine
	clinical pharmacokinetic service
	coagulase-positive staphylococci
	complex partial seizures
CPT	chest physiotherapy
	child protection team
	Continuous Performance Test
CPTA	Certified Physical Therapy Assistant
CPTH	chronic post-traumatic headache
CPUE	chest pain of unknown etiology
CPX	complete physical examination
CPZ	chlorpromazine
	Compazine® (CPZ is a dangerous abbreviation as it could be either)
CQI	continuous quality improvement
CR	cardiac rehabilitation
	cardiorespiratory
	case reports
	chief resident
	closed reduction
	colon resection
	complete remission
	contact record
	controlled release
	creamed
	cycloplegia retinoscopy
Cr	chromium

C & R	cystoscopy and retrograde
CR$_1$	first cranial nerve
CRA	central retinal artery
	chronic rheumatoid arthritis
	colorectal anastomosis
CRAG	cerebral radionuclide angiography
CrAg	cryptococcal antigen
CRAMS	circulation, respiration, abdomen, motor, and speech
CRAN	craniotomy
CRAO	central retinal artery occlusion
CRBBB	complete right bundle branch block
CRBP	cellular retinol-binding protein
CRC	Certified Research Coordinator
	child-resistant container
	clinical research center
	colorectal cancer
CR & C	closed reduction and cast
CrCl	creatinine clearance
CRD	childhood rheumatic disease
	chronic renal disease
	chronic respiratory disease
	cone-rod dystrophy
	congenital rubella deafness
CREAT	serum creatinine
CREST	calcinosis, Raynaud's disease, esophageal dysmotility, sclerodactyly, and telangiectasia
CRF	chronic renal failure
	corticotropin-releasing factor
CRFZ	closed reduction of fractured zygoma
CRI	Cardiac Risk Index
	catheter-related infection
	chronic renal insufficiency

CRIE	crossed radioimmuno-electrophoresis	
CRIF	closed reduction and internal fixation	
crit.	hematocrit	
CRL	crown rump length	
CRM	cream	
CRM +	cross-reacting material positive	
CRNA	Certified Registered Nurse Anesthetist	
CRNI	Certified Registered Nurse Intravenous	
CRNP	Certified Registered Nurse Practitioner	
CRO	cathode ray oscilloscope	
	contract research organizations(s)	
CROS	contralateral routing of signals	
CRP	chronic relapsing pancreatitis	
	coronary rehabilitation program	
	C-reactive protein	
C&RP	curettage and root planning	
CRPD	chronic restrictive pulmonary disease	
CRPF	chloroquine-resistant *Plasmodium falciparum*	
CRQ	Chronic Respiratory (Disease) Questionnaire	
CRS	Carroll Self-Rating Scale	
	catheter-related sepsis	
	Chinese restaurant syndrome	
	colon-rectal surgery	
	congenital rubella syndrome	
	cryoreductive surgery	
CRST	calcification, Raynaud's phenomenom, scleroderma, and telangiectasia	
CRT	cadaver renal transplant	
	cathode ray tube	
	central reaction time	
	copper reduction test	

	cranial radiation therapy
Cr Tr	crutch training
CRTT	Certified Respiratory Therapy Technician
CRTX	cast removed take x-ray
CRU	cardiac rehabilitation unit
	clinical research unit
CRV	central retinal vein
CRVF	congestive right ventricular failure
CRVO	central retinal vein occlusion
CRYST	crystals
CS	cat scratch
	cervical spine
	cesarean section
	chest strap
	cholesterol stone
	cigarette smoker
	clinical stage
	close supervision
	conjunctiva-sclera
	consciousness
	consultation
	consultation service
	coronary sinus
	Cushing's syndrome
	cycloserine
C&S	conjunctiva and sclera
	cough and sneeze
	culture and sensitivity
C/S	cesarean section
	culture and sensitivity
CSA	compressed spectral activity
	controlled substance analogue
CsA	cyclosporin
CSB	caffeine sodium benzoate
	Cheyne-Stokes breathing
	Children's Services Board
CSB I & II	Chemistry Screening Batteries I and II
CSBF	coronary sinus blood flow
CSC	cornea, sclera, and conjunctiva
CSCI	continuous subcutaneous infusion
CSCR	central serous chorioretinopathy

CSD	cat scratch disease	
C S&D	cleaned, sutured, and dressed	
CSE	cross-section echocardiography	
C sect.	cesarean section	
CSF	cerebrospinal fluid	
	colony-stimulating factors	
CSFP	cerebrospinal fluid pressure	
C-Sh	chair shower	
CSH	carotid sinus hypersensitivity	
	chronic subdural hematoma	
CSI	Computerized Severity Index	
	continuous subcutaneous infusion	
CSICU	cardiac surgery intensive care unit	
CSII	continuous subcutaneous insulin infusion	
CS IV	clinical stage 4	
CSLU	chronic status leg ulcer	
CSM	carotid sinus massage	
	cerebrospinal meningitis	
	circulation, sensation, and movement	
CSME	cotton spot macular edema	
CSMN	chronic sensorimotor neuropathy	
CSN	cystic suppurative necrosis	
CSNRT	corrected sinus node recovery time	
CSNS	carotid sinus nerve stimulation	
CSO	copied standing orders	
CSOM	chronic serous otitis media	
	chronic suppurative otitis media	
CSP	cellulose sodium phosphate	
CSR	central supply room	
	Cheyne-Strokes respiration	

corrective septorhinoplasty

CSS carotid sinus stimulation
Central Sterile Services
chewing, sucking, and
swallowing

C_{ss} concentration of drug at
steady-state

CSSD closed system sterile
drainage

CST cardiac stress test
cerebroside sulfotrans-
ferase
Certified Surgical
Technologist
contraction stress test
convulsive shock therapy
cosyntropin stimulation
test
static compliance

C_{STAT} static lung compliance

CSU cardiac surgery unit
cardiac surveillance unit
cardiovascular surgery
unit
casualty staging unit
catheter specimen of urine

CT calcitonin
cardiothoracic
carpal tunnel
cervical traction
chemotherapy
chest tube
circulation time
clotting time
coagulation time
coated tablet
compressed tablet
computed tomography
Coomb's test
corneal thickness
corneal transplant
corrective therapy
cytarabine and
thioguanine
cytoxic drug

C_t concentration of drug in
tissue

CTA catamenia (menses)
clear to auscultation

C-TAB	cyanide tablet		carpal tunnel repair
CTAP	clear to auscultation and percussion	CTRS	Conners Teachers Rating Scale
	computed tomography during arterial portography	CTS	carpal tunnel syndrome
		CTSP	called to see patient
CTB	ceased to breathe	CTW	central terminal of Wilson
CTC	circular tear capsulotomy	CTX	cerebrotendinous xanthomatosis
CTCL	cutaneous T-cell lymphoma		cyclophosphamide (Cytoxan®)
CT & DB	cough, turn & deep breath	CTXN	contraction
CTD	carpal tunnel decompression	CTZ	chemoreceptor trigger zone
	chest tube drainage		co-trimoxazole (sulfamethoxazole-trimethoprin)
	connective tissue disease		
	corneal thickness depth	Cu	copper
CTDW	continues to do well	CU	cause unknown
CTF	Colorado tick fever	CUC	chronic ulcerative colitis
	continuous tube feeding		Clinical Unit Clerk
C/TG	cholesterol to triglyceride ratio	CUD	cause undetermined
		CUG	cystourethrogram
CTGA	complete transposition of the great arteries	CUP	carcinoma of unknown primary (site)
	corrected transposition of the great arteries	CUPS	carcinoma of unknown primary site
CTH	clot to hold	CUR	curettage
CTI	certification of terminal illness		cystourethrorectocele
CTL	cervical, thoracic, and lumbar	CUS	chronic undifferentiated schizophrenia
			contact urticaria syndrome
	chronic tonsillitis	CUSA	Cavitron ultrasonic suction aspirator
	cytotoxic T-lymphocytes		
CTM	Chlor-Trimeton®	CUT	chronic undifferentiated type (schizophrenia)
	clinical trials materials		
CT/MPR	computed tomography with multiplanar reconstructions	CV	cardiovascular
			cell volume
			cisplatin and etoposide
CTN	calcitonin		coefficient of variation
C & T N, BLE	color and temperature normal, both lower extremities		color vision
			common ventricle
			consonant vowel
cTNM	clinical-diagnostic staging of cancer	CVA	cerebrovascular accident
			costovertebral angle
CTP	comprehensive treatment plan	CVAH	congenital virilizing adrenal hyperplasia
CTPN	central total parenteral nutrition	CVAT	costovertebral angle tenderness
CTR	carpal tunnel release	CVB	group B coxsackievirus

CVC	central venous catheter		prednisone
	consonant vowel consonant	CVR	cerebral vascular resistance
CVD	cardiovascular disease	CVRI	coronary vascular resistance index
	collagen vascular disease		
CVEB	cisplatin, vinblastine, etoposide, and bleomycin	CVS	cardiovascular surgery chorionic villi sampling clean voided specimen
CVF	cardiovascular failure	CVSCU	cardiovascular special care unit
	central visual field		
	cervicovaginal fluid	CVSU	cardiovascular specialty unit
CVG	coronary vein graft		
CVHD	chronic valvular heart disease	CVTC	central venous tunneled catheter
CVI	carboplatin, etoposide, ifosfamide, and mesna uroprotection	CVU	clean voided urine
		CVUG	cysto-void urethrogram
		CW	careful watch
	cerebrovascular insufficiency		chest wall
			clockwise
	common variable immunodeficiency (disease)		compare with
		C/W	consistent with
			crutch walking
	continuous venous infusion	CWAF	Chemical Withdrawal Assessment Flowsheet
CVICU	cardiovascular intensive care unit	CWD	cell wall defective
		CWE	cotton wool exudates
CVID	common variable immune deficiency	CWL	Caldwell-Luc
CVINT	cardiovascular intermediate	CWMS	color, warmth, movement, and sensation
CVL	central venous line	CWP	centimeters of water pressure
CVMT	cervical-vaginal, motion tenderness		childbirth without pain
CVN	central venous nutrient		coal worker's pneumoconiosis
CVNSR	cardiovascular normal sinus rhythm		
CVO	central vein occlusion	CWS	comfortable walking speed
	conjugate diameter of pelvic inlet		cotton wool spots
CvO_2	mixed venous oxygen content	Cx	cancel
			cervix
			culture
CVOR	cardiovascular operating room		cylinder axis
		CXA	circumflex artery
CVP	central venous pressure	CxBx	cervical biopsy
	cyclophosphamide, vincristine, and prednisone	CxMT	cervical motion tenderness
		CXR	chest x-ray
		CXTX	cervical traction
CVPP	lomustine, vinblastine, procarbazine, and	CY	cyclophosphamide

CYA	cover your ass
CyA	cyclosporine
CyADIC	cyclophosphamide, doxorubicin, and dacarbazine
Cyclo C	cyclocytidine HCl
CYL	cylinder
CYP	cytochrome P-450
CYSTO	cystogram
	cystoscopy
CYT	cyclophosphamide
CYVA DIC	cyclophosphamide, vincristine, Adriamycin®, and dacarbazine
CZE	capillary zone electrophoresis
CZI	crystalline zinc insulin (regular insulin)
CZN	chlorzotocin

D

D	daughter
	day
	dead
	depression
	dextrose
	diarrhea
	diastole
	dilated
	diopter
	distal
	distance
	divorced
D-1 to D-12	dorsal vertebrae 1 to 12
D_2	ergocalciferol
D_3	cholecalciferol
D50	50% dextrose injection
2/d	twice a day (this is a dangerous abbreviation)
2-D	two-dimensional
3-D	three-dimensional

4D	4 prism diopters
DA	degenerative arthritis
	delivery awareness
	Dental Assistant
	diagnostic arthroscopy
	direct admission
	direct agglutination
	dopamine
	drug addict
	drug aerosol
D/A	discharge and advise
DA/A	drug/alcohol addiction
DAB	days after birth
DAC	day activity center
	disabled adult child
	Division of Ambulatory Care
DACL	Depression Adjective Checklists
DACT	dactinomycin
DAD	diffuse alveolar damage
	dispense as directed
	drug administration device
DAE	diving air embolism
DAG	diacylglyerol
	dianhydrogalactitol
DAH	disordered action of the heart
DAI	diffuse axonal injury
DAL	drug analysis laboratory
DAM	diacetylmonoxine
DANA	drug induced antinuclear antibodies
DAo	descending aorta
DAP	draw a person
	diabetes-associated peptide
	diastolic augmentation pressure
DAR	daily affective rhythm
DARE	data, action, response, and evaluation
DARP	drug abuse rehabilitation program
	drug abuse reporting program
DAS	developmental apraxia of speech

	died at scene		diagonal conjugate
DAT	daunorubicin, cytarabine, (ARA-C), and thioguanine		direct Coombs (test)
			discharged
			discontinue
	dementia of the Alzheimer type	DC65®	Darvon Compound 65®
		DCA	sodium dichloroacetate
	diet as tolerated	DCAG	double coronary artery graft
	diphtheria antitoxin		
	direct agglutination test	DCBE	double contrast barium enema
	direct antiglobulin test		
DAU	drug abuse urine	DCC	day care center
DAUNO	daunorubicin	DCCF	dural carotid-cavernous fistula
DAVA	vindesine sulfate		
DAW	dispense as written	DCCT	Diabetes Control and Complications Trial (questionnaire)
DAWN	Drug Abuse Warning Network		
dB	decibel		
DB	date of birth	DCE	delayed contrast-enhancement
	deep breathe		
	demonstration bath		designated compensable event
	direct bilirubin		
	double blind	DCF	data collection form
DB & C	deep breathing and coughing		pentostatin (deoxyco-formycin)
DBD	milolactol (dibromodulici-tol)	DCFS	Department of Children and Family Services
DBE	deep breathing exercise	DCH	delayed cutaneous hypersensitivity
DBED	penicillin G benzathine		
D₅BES	dextrose in balanced electrolyte solution	DCIS	ductal carcinoma *in situ*
		DCM	dilated cardiomyopathy
DBI®	phenformin HCl	DCMXT	dichloromethotrexate
DBIL	direct bilirubin	DCN	Darvocet N®
DBL	double beta-lactam	DCNU	chlorozotocin
DBP	D-binding protein	DCO	diffusing capacity of carbon monoxide
	diastolic blood pressure		
DBPT	dacarbazine (DTIC), carmustine (BCNU), cisplatin (Platinol), and tamoxifen	DCP	dynamic compression plate
		DCP®	calcium phosphate, dibasic
DBQ	debrisoquin	DCPM	daunorubicin, cytarabine, prednisolone, and mercaptopurine
DBS	diminished breath sounds		
DBZ	dibenzamine	DCPN	direction-changing positional nystagmus
DC	daunorubicin and cytarabine		
	dextrocardia	DCR	dacryocystorhinostomy
	Doctor of Chiropractic		delayed cutaneous reaction
D&C	dilation and curettage	DCS	decompression sickness
	direct and consensual		dorsal column stimulator
d/c, DC	decrease	DCSA	double contrast shoulder arthrography

DCT	daunorubicin, cytarabine, and thioguanine	D_5E_{48}	5% Dextrose and Electrolyte 48
	deep chest therapy	D_5E_{75}	5% Dextrose and Electrolyte 75
	direct (antiglobulin) Coombs test	2DE	two-dimensional echocardiography
DCTM	delay computer tomographic myelography	D&E	dilation and evacuation
		DEA#	Drug Enforcement Administration number (physician's Federal narcotic number)
DCU	day care unit		
DCYS	Department of Children and Youth Services		
DD	dependent drainage	DEB	dystrophic epidermolysis bullosa
	dialysis dementia		
	died of the disease	DEC	decrease
	differential diagnosis		diethylcarbamazine
	discharge diagnosis	DECA	nandrolone decanoate
	disk diameter	DECAFS	Department of Children and Family Services
	down drain		
	dry dressing	DECEL	deceleration
	Duchenne's dystrophy	decub	decubitus
D/D	diarrhea/dehydration	DEEDS	drugs, exercise, education, diet, and self-monitoring
D→D	discharge to duty		
D & D	diarrhea and dehydration		
DDA	dideoxyadenosine	DEEG	deteriorating electroencephalogram
DDAVP®	desmopressin acetate		
DDC	zalcitabine (dideoxycytidine)	DEET	diethyltoluamide
		DEF	decayed, extracted, or filled
DDD	defined daily doses		defecation
	degenerative disc disease		deficiency
	fully automatic pacing	degen	degenerative
DDGB	double-dose gallbladder (test)	del	delivery, delivered
		DEM	drug evaluation matrix
DDHT	double dissociated hypertropia	DEP ST SEG	depressed ST segment
DDI	didanosine (dideoxyinosine)	DER	disulfiram-ethanol reaction
DDP	cisplatin	DERM	dermatology
DDS	dialysis disequilibrium syndrome	DES	diethylstilbestrol
	Doctor of Dental Surgery		diffuse esophageal spasm
	double decidual sac (sign)		disequilibrium syndrome
	4, 4-diaminodiphenyl-sulfone (dapsone)		dry eye syndrome
		DESAT	desaturation
DDST	Denver Development Screening Test	DESI	Drug Efficacy Study Implementation (Project)
DDT	chlorophenothane		
DDTP	drug dependence treatment program	DET	diethyltryptamine
		DEV	deviation
DDx	differential diagnosis		duck embryo vaccine

DEVR	dominant exudative vitreoretinopathy	D+H	delusions and hallucinations
dex.	dexter (right)	DHA	dihydroxyacetone
DF	decayed and filled		docosahexaenoic acid
	degree of freedom	DHAC	dihydro-5-azacytidine
	dengue fever	DHAD	mitoxanthrone HCl
	diabetic father	DHBV	duck hepatitis B virus
	diastolic filling	DHCA	deep hypothermia circulatory arrest
	dorsiflexion		
	drug free	DHCC	dihydroxycholecalciferol
	dye free	DHE 45®	dihydroergotamine mesylate
DFA	diet for age		
	difficulty falling asleep	DHEA	dehydroepiandrosterone
	direct fluorescent antibody	DHEAS	dehydroepiandrosterone sulfate
DFD	defined formula diets	DHF	dengue hemorrhagic fever
	degenerative facet disease	DHFR	dihydrofolate reductase
DFE	dilated fundus examination	DHL	diffuse histocytic lymphoma
	distal femoral epiphysis	DHPG	ganciclovir
DFG	direct forward gaze	DHPR	erythrocyte dihydropteri-dine reductase
DFI	disease-free interval		
DFM	decreased fetal movement	DHS	Department of Human Services
DFMC	daily fetal movement count		duration of hospital stay
DFMO	eflornithine (difluoro-methylorithine)		dynamic hip screw
		DHST	delayed hypersensitivity test
DFMR	daily fetal movement record	DHT	dihydrotachysterol
DFO	deferoxamine		dihydrotestosterone
DFOM	deferoxamine		dissociated hypertropia
DFP	diastolic filling period		Dobbhoff tube
	isoflurophate (diisopropyl flurophosphate)	DI	(Beck) Depression Inventory
DFR	diabetic floor routine		date of injury
DFRC	deglycerolized frozen red cells		Debrix Index
			detrusor instability
DFS	disease-free survival		diabetes insipidus
DFU	dead fetus in uterus		diagnostic imaging
DFW	Dexide face wash		drug interactions
DGE	delayed gastric emptying	D&I	debridement and irrigation
DGI	disseminated gonococcal infection		dry and intact
		diag.	diagnosis
DGM	ductal glandular mastectomy	DIAS BP	diastolic blood pressure
		Diath SW	diathermy short wave
DH	delayed hypersensitivity	DIAZ	diazepam
	dermatitis herpetiformis	DIB	disability insurance benefits
	developmental history		
	diaphragmatic hernia	DIC	dacarbazine

	differential interference contrast	DIS	Diagnostic Interview Schedule (questionnaire)
	disseminated intravascular coagulation		dislocation
	drug information center	disch.	discharge
DICC	dynamic infusion cavernosometry and cavernosography	DISH	diffuse idiopathic skeletal hyperostosis
DICLOX	dicloxacillin	DISI	dorsal intercalated segmental (segment) instability
DICP	demyelinated inflammatory chronic polyneuropathy	D₅ISOM	5% Dextrose and Isolyte M
DID	delayed ischemia deficit	D₅ISOP	5% Dextrose and Isolyte P
DIE	die in emergency department	dist.	distal
			distilled
DIF	differentiation-inducing factor	DIT	diiodotyrosine
DIFF	differential blood count		drug-induced thrombocytopenia
DIG	digoxin (this is a dangerous abbreviation)	DIU	death in utero
DIH	died in hospital	DIV	double inlet ventricle
DIJOA	dominantly inherited juvenile optic atrophy	DIVA	digital intravenous angiography
DIL	daughter-in-law	Div ex	divergence excess
	dilute	DJD	degenerative joint disease
	drug-induced lupus	DK	dark
DILD	diffuse infiltrative lung disease		diabetic ketoacidosis
			diseased kidney
DILE	drug induced lupus erythematosus	DKA	diabetic ketoacidosis
			didn't keep appointment
DIM	diminish	dl	deciliter (100 mL)
DIMD	drug induced movement disorders	DL	danger list
			deciliter
DIMOAD	diabetes insipidus, diabetes mellitus, optic atrophy, and deafness		diagnostic laparoscopy
			direct laryngoscopy
			drug level
DIMS	disorders of initiating and maintaining sleep	D_L	maximal diffusing capacity
DIOS	distal intestinal obstruction syndrome	DLB	direct laryngoscopy and bronchoscopy
DIP	desquamative interstitial pneumonia	DLC	diffuse large cell
			double lumen catheter
	diplopia	DLCO sb	diffusion capacity of carbon monoxide, single breath
	distal interphalangeal		
	drip infusion pyelogram		
	drug-induced parkinsonism	DLD	date of last drink
DIPJ	distal interphalangeal joint	DLE	discoid lupus erythematosus
DIR	directions	DLF	digitalis-like factor

DLIF	digoxin-like immunoreactive factors	DMI	desipramine
			diaphragmatic myocardial infarction
DLIS	digoxin-like immunoreactive substance	DMKA	diabetes mellitus ketoacidosis
DLMP	date of last menstrual period	DMO	dimethadone
DLNG	dl-norgestrel	DMOOC	diabetes mellitus out of control
DLNMP	date of last normal menstrual period	DMP	dimethyl phthalate
D5LR	dextrose 5% in lactated Ringer's injection	DMSA	dimercaptosuccinic acid
		DMSO	dimethyl sulfoxide
DLPD	diffuse lymphocytic poorly differentiated	DMT	dimethyltryptamine
DLS	daily living skills	DMV	Doctor of Veterinary Medicine
DLSC	double lumen subclavian catheter	DMX	diathermy, massage, and exercise
DLT	double-lung transplant	DN	diabetic nephropathy
DM	dehydrated and malnourished		dicrotic notch
			down
	dermatomyositis		dysplastic nevus
	dextromethorphan	D & N	distance and near (vision)
	diabetes mellitus	D5NS	dextrose 5% in 0.9% sodium chloride injection
	diabetic mother		
	diastolic murmur		
DMAD	disease-modifying antirheumatic drug	D₅ 1/2NS	dextrose 5% in 0.45% sodium chloride injection
DMARD	disease modifying antirheumatic drug	DNA	deoxyribonucleic acid
			did not answer
DMAS	Drug Management and Authorization Section		did not attend
			does not apply
DMBA	dimethylbenzanthracene	DNCB	dinitrochlorobenzene
DMC	dactinomycin, methotrexate, and cyclophosphamide	DNC	did not come
		DND	died a natural death
		DNFC	does not follow commands
	diabetes management center	DNI	do not intubate
DMD	disciform macular degeneration	DNIC	diffuse noxious inhibitory control
	Doctor of Dental Medicine	DNKA	did not keep appointment
		DNP	dinitrophenylhydrazine
	Duchenne's muscular dystrophy		do not publish
DMD w/ SRNM	disciform macular degeneration with subretinal neovascular membrane	DNR	daunorubicin
			did not respond
			do not report
			do not resuscitate
			dorsal nerve root
DME	durable medical equipment	DNS	deviated nasal septum
DMF	decayed, missing, or filled		doctor did not see patient

	do not show	DOSS	docusate sodium (dioctyl sodium sulfosuccinate)
	dysplastic nevus syndrome	DOT	date of transcription
D₅NSS	5% dextrose in normal saline solution		date of transfer
			died on table
DNT	did not test		Doppler ophthalmic test
DO	diet order	DOX	doxepin
	distocclusal		doxorubicin
	Doctor of Osteopathy	doz	dozen
	doctor's order	DP	diastolic pressure
D/O	disorder		disability pension
✔DO	check doctor's order		discharge planning
DO₂	oxygen delivery		dorsalis pedis (pulse)
DOA	date of admission	DPA	Department of Public Assistance
	dead on arrival		dipropylacetic acid
	duration of action		dual photon absorptiometry
DOA-DRA	dead on arrival despite resuscitative attempts		durable power of attorney
DOB	dangle out of bed	DPAP	diastolic pulmonary artery pressure
	date of birth		
	dobutamine	DPB	days postburn
	doctor's order book	DPC	delayed primary closure
DOC	date of conception		discharge planning coordinator
	diabetes out of control		
	died of other causes	DPDL	diffuse poorly differentiated lymphocytic lymphoma
	diet of choice		
	drug of choice		
DOCA	desoxycorticosterone acetate	2.3-DPG	2,3-diphosphoglyceric acid
DOD	date of death	DPH	Department of Public Health
DOE	dyspnea on exertion		
DOES	disorders of excessive somnolence		diphenhydramine
			Doctor of Public Health
DOH	Department of Health		phenytoin (diphenylhydantoin)
DOI	date of implant (pacemaker)		
		DPL	diagnostic peritoneal lavage
	date of injury		
DOL	days of life	D5PLM	dextrose 5% and Plasmalyte M® injection
DOL #2	second day of life		
DOLV	double outlet left ventricle		
DOM	Doctor of Oriental Medicine	DPM	distintegrations per minute (dpm)
	domiciliary care		Doctor of Podiatric Medicine
DON	Director of Nursing		
DOP	dopamine		drops per minute
DORV	double-outlet right ventricle	DPN	diabetic peripheral neuropathy
DORx	date of treatment		
DOSA	day of surgery admission	DPP	dorsalis pedal pulse

DPPC	colfosceril palmitate (dipalmitoylphosphatidylcholine)	D/S	5% dextrose and 0.9% sodium chloride injection
DPT	Demerol®, Phenergan®, and Thorazine® (this is a dangerous abbreviation)	D&S	diagnostic and surgical dilation and suction
	diphtheria, pertussis, and tetanus (immunization)	D5S	dextrose 5% in 0.9% sodium chloride (saline) injection
	Driver Performance Test	DSA	digital subtraction angiography (angiocardiography)
DPTPM	diphtheria, pertussis, tetanus, poliomyelitis, and measles	DSB	drug-seeking behavior
DPU	delayed pressure urticaria	DSD	discharge summary dictated
DPUD	duodenal peptic ulcer disease		dry sterile dressing
DPVSs	dilated perivascular spaces	DSDB	direct self-destructive behavior
D&Q	deep and quiet	dsg	dressing
Dr.	doctor	DSI	deep shock insulin
DR	delivery room		Depression Status Inventory
	diabetic retinopathy	DSM	drink skim milk
	diagnostic radiology	DSM III	Diagnostic & Statistical Manual, 3rd Edition
	diurnal rhythm		
DRA	drug-related admissions	DSP	digital signal processor
DRAPE	drug-related adverse patient event	D-SPINE	dorsal spine
		DSRF	drainage subretinal fluid
DRE	digital rectal examination	DSS	dengue shock syndrome
DRESS	depth resolved surface coil spectroscopy		Disability Status Scale
			docusate sodium
DREZ	dorsal root entry zone	DSST	Digit-Symbol Substitution Test
DRG	diagnosis-related groups		
DRGE	drainage	DST	donor-specific (blood) transfusion
drI	Discharge Readiness Index		
		DSU	day stay unit
DRM	drug-related morbidity		day surgery unit
DRP	drug-related problem	DSV	digital subtraction ventriculography
DRS	Duane's retraction syndrome		
		DSWI	deep surgical wound infection
DRSG	dressing	DT	delirium tremens
DRUB	drug screen-blood		dietetic technician
DRUJ	distal or radial ulnar joint		diphtheria tetanus
DS	deep sleep		diphtheria toxoid
	Dextrostix®		discharge tomorrow
	discharge summary	D/T	due to
	disoriented	D&T	diagnosis and treatment
	double strength	DTBC	tubocurarine (D-tubocurarine)
	Down's syndrome		
	drug screen		

DTBE	Division of Tuberculosis Elimination	DUSN	diffuse unilateral subacute neuroretinitis
DTC	day treatment center diticarb (diethyldiothio-carbamate) tubocurarine (D-tubocurarine)	DV	distance vision
		D&V	diarrhea and vomiting
		DVA	distance visual acuity vindesine
DTD #30	dispense 30 such doses	DVC	direct visualization of vocal cords
DTH	delayed-type hypersensitivity	D V® Cream	dienestrol vaginal cream
DTIC	dacarbazine	DVD	dissociated vertical deviation double vessel disease
DTO	deodorized tincture of opium (warning: this is *NOT* paregoric)	DVI	atrioventricular sequential pacing digital vascular imaging
DTOGV	dextral-transposition of great vessels		
DTPA	pentetic acid (diethylenetriaminepen-taacetic acid)	DVIU	direct vision internal urethrotomy
		DVM	Doctor of Veterinary Medicine
DTR	deep tendon reflexes	DVP	cyclophosphamide, vincristine, and prednisone
DTs	delirium tremens		
DTS	donor specific transfusion		
DTT	diphtheria tetanus toxoid dithiothreitol	DVP-Asp	daunorubicin, vincristine, prednisone, and asparaginase
DTUS	diathermy, traction, and ultrasound		
DTV	due to void	DVPA	daunorubicin, vincristine, prednisone, and asparaginase
DTX	detoxification		
DU	diabetic urine diagnosis undetermined duodenal ulcer duroxide uptake	DVR	Division of Vocational Rehabilitation double valve replacement
DUB	Dubowitz (score) dysfunctional uterine bleeding	DVSA	digital venous subtraction angiography
		DVT	deep vein thrombosis
DUI	driving under the influence	DVTS	deep venous thromboscintigram
DUID	driving under the influence of drugs	DVVC	direct visualization of vocal cords
DUII	driving under the influence of intoxicants	DW	deionized water dextrose in water distilled water doing well
DUIL	driving under the influence of liquor		
DUN	dialysate urea nitrogen	D_5W	5% dextrose (in water) injection
DUNHL	diffuse undifferentiated non-Hodgkins lymphoma	D10W	10% dextrose (in water) injection
DUR	drug use review duration	D20W	20% dextrose (in water) injection

D50W	50% dextrose (in water) injection			auscultation of lung showing consolidation
D70W	70% dextrose (in water) injection	EA	elbow aspiration
			enteral alimentation
5 DW	5% dextrose (in water) injection	E&A	evaluate and advise
		EAA	electrothermal atomic absorption
DWDL	diffuse well differentiated lymphocytic lymphoma		essential amino acids
			excitatory amino acid
DWI	driving while intoxicated	EAB	elective abortion
DWRT	delayed work recall test	EAC	external auditory canal
Dx	diagnosis	EACA	aminocaproic acid
DXM	dexamethasone	EAHF	eczema, allergy, and hay fever
DXRT	deep x-ray therapy		
DXS	Dextrostix®	EAM	external auditory meatus
DY	dysprosium	EAP	Employment Assistance Programs
DYF	drag your feet (author's note: see you in court)		
		EAS	external anal sphincter
DYFS	Division of Youth and Family Services	EAST	external rotation, abduction stress test
DZ	diazepam	EAT	Eating Attitudes Test
	disease		ectopic atrial tachycardia
	dizygotic	EAU	experimental autoimmune uveitis
	dozen		
DZP	diazepam	EB	epidermolysis bullosa
			Epstein-Barr
		EBA	epidermolysis bullosa acquisita
	E	EBAB	equal breath sounds bilaterally
		EBC	esophageal balloon catheter
		EBEA	Epstein-Barr (virus) early antigen
E	edema	EBF	erythroblastosis fetalis
	eloper	EBL	estimated blood loss
	engorged	EBM	expressed breast milk
	eosinophil	EBNA	Epstein-Barr (virus) nuclear antigen
	esophoria for distance		
	evaluation	EBP	epidural blood patch
	expired	EBS	epidermolysis bullosa
	eye	EBSB	equal breath sounds bilaterally
E'	esophoria for near		
E_1	estrone	EBV	Epstein-Barr virus
E2	estradiol	EBVCA	Epstein-Barr viral capsid antigen
E3	estriol		
4E	4 plus edema	EBVEA	Epstein-Barr virus, early antigen
E20	Enfamil 20®		
E→A	say E,E,E, comes out as A,A,A upon	EBVNA	Epstein-Barr virus, nuclear antigen

EC	ejection click	ECM/	extracellular mass, body
	enteric coated	BCM	cell mass ratio
	Escherichia coli	ECMO	extracorporeal membrane
	extracellular		oxygenation
	eyes closed		(oxygenator)
ECA	Epidemiological	ECN	extended care nursery
	Catchment Area	ECochG	electrocochleography
	ethacrynic acid	ECOG	Eastern Cooperative
	external carotid artery		Oncology Group
ECBD	exploration of common	ECoG	electrocochleography
	bile duct		electrocorticogram
ECC	emergency cardiac care	ECP	extracorporeal
	endocervical curettage		photochemotherapy
	external cardiac	ECPD	external counterpressure
	compression		device
	extracorporeal circulation	ECR	emergency chemical
ECCE	extracapsular cataract		restraint
	extraction		extensor carpi radialis
ECD	endocardial cushion	ECRB	extensor carpi radialis
	defect		brevis
ECEMG	evoked compound	ECRL	extensor carpi radialis
	electromyography		longus
ECF	extended care facility	ECS	electrocerebral silence
	extracellular fluid	ECT	electroconvulsive therapy
ECF-A	eosinophil chemotactic		emission computed
	factors of anaphylaxis		tomography
ECG	electrocardiogram		enhanced computed
ECHINO	echinocyte		tomography
ECHO	echocardiogram	ECU	electrocautery unit
	enterocytopathogenic		extensor carpi ulnaris
	human orphan (virus)	ECV	external cephalic version
	etoposide, cyclophospha-	ECW	extracellular water
	mide, Adriamycin®,	ED	elbow disarticulation
	and vincristine		emergency department
			epidural
ECHO/	echocardiography/radionu-		ethynodiol diacetate
RV	clide ventriculography	ED_{50}	median effective dose
ECI	extracorporeal irradiation	EDAP	Emergency Department
ECIB	extracorporeal irradiation		Approved for Pediatrics
	of blood	EDAS	encephalodural
ECIC	extracranial to intracranial		arterio-synangiosis
	(anastamosis)	EDAT	Emergency Department
EC/IC	extracranial/intracranial		Alert Team
ECL	extend of cerebral lesion	EDAX	energy-dispersive analysis
	extracapillary lesions		of x-rays
ECM	erythema chronicum	EDB	ethylene dibromide
	migrans		extensor digitorum brevis
	extracellular mass	EDC	effective dynamic
	extracellular matrix		compliance

	electrodesiccation and curettage	Syndrome	dysplasia, cleft syndrome
	end diastolic counts	EEE	Eastern equine encephalomyelitis
	estimated date of conception		edema, erythema, and exudate
	estimated date of confinement		external eye examination
	extensor digitorium communis	EEG	electroencephalogram
EDCP	eccentric dynamic compression plates	EENT	eyes, ears, nose, and throat
EDD	expected date of delivery	EEP	end expiratory pressure
EDENT	edentulous	EES®	erythromycin ethylsuccinate
EDF	elongation, derotation, and flexion	EEV	encircling endocardial ventriculotomy
EDH	epidural hematoma	EF	ejection fraction
EDI	Eating Disorders Inventory		endurance factor
			erythroblastosis fetalis
EDITAR	extended-duration topical arthropod repellent		extended-field (radiotherapy)
EDM	early diastolic murmur	EFAD	essential fatty acid deficiency
EDP	emergency department physician	EFE	endocardial fibroelastosis
	end diastolic pressure	EFF	effacement
EDQ	extensor digiti quinti (tendon)	EFS	event-free survival
EDQV	extensor digiti quinti five	EFHBM	eosinophilic fibrohistiocytic lesion of bone marrow
EDR	edrophonium		
EDRF	endothelium derived relaxing factor	EFM	electronic fetal monitor(ing)
EDS	Ehlers-Danlos syndrome		external fetal monitoring
	excessive daytime somnolence	EFN	effusion
EDTA	edetic acid (ethylenediaminetetraacetic acid)	EFW	estimated fetal weight
		EF/WM	ejection fraction/wall motion
EDV	end-diastolic volume	e.g.	for example
	epidermal dysplastic verruciformis	EGA	esophageal gastric (tube) airway
EDW	estimated dry weight		estimated gestational age
EE	end to end	EGBUS	external genitalia, Bartholin, urethral, and Skene's glands
	equine encephalitis		
	external ear		
	eye and ear	EGC	early gastric carcinoma
EEA	electroencephalic audiometry	EGFR	epidermal growth factor receptor
	elemental enteral alimentation	EGD	esophagogastroduodenoscopy
	end-to-end anastomosis	EGF	epidermal growth factor
EEC	ectrodactyly-ectodermal	EGG	electrogastrography

EGJ	esophagogastric junction	EKG	electrocardiogram
EGL	eosinophilic granuloma of the lung	EKO	echoencephalogram
		EKY	electrokymogram
EGTA	esophageal gastric tube airway	E-L	external lids
		ELF	elective low forceps
EH	educationally handicapped	ELH	endolymphatic hydrops
	enlarged heart	ELI	endomyocardial lymphocytic infiltrates
	essential hypertension		
	extramedullary hematopoiesis	ELISA	enzyme-linked immunosorbent assay
EHB	elevate head of bed	Elix	elixir
	extensor hallucis brevis	ELLIP	elliptocytosis
EHBA	extrahepatic biliary atresia	ELMA	endothelial leukocyte adhesion molecule
EHDA	etidronate sodium		
EHDP	etidronate disodium	ELO	enteroviral leukemic oncogene
EHE	epithelioid hemangioen- dothelioma		
		ELOP	estimated length of program
EHEC	enterohemorrhagic *Escherichia coli*		
		ELOS	estimated length of stay
EHF·	epidemic hemorrhagic fever	ELP	electrophoresis
		ELPS	excessive lateral pressure syndrome
EHL	electrohydraulic lithotripsy		
		ELS	Eaton-Lambert syndrome
	extensor hallucis longus	ELT	euglobulin lysis time
E & I	endocrine and infertility	EM	early memory
EIA	enzyme immunoassay		ejection murmur
	exercise induced asthma		electron microscope
EIAB	extracranial-intracranial arterial bypass		emmetropia
			erythema migrans
EIB	exercise induced bronchospasm		erythema multiforme
			extensive metabolizers
EID	electroimmunodiffusion	EMA	early morning awakening
	electronic infusion device		endomysial antibody
EIEC	enteroinvasive *Escherichia coli*	EMA-CO	etoposide, methotrexate, dactinomycin, and leucovorin
EIP	elective interruption of pregnancy		
		EMB	endometrial biopsy
	end-inspiratory pressure		endomyocardial biopsy
	extensor indicis proprius		ethambutol
EIS	endoscopic injection scleropathy	EMC	encephalomyocarditis
		EMD	electromechanical dissociation
EJ	elbow jerk		
	external jugular	EMDR	eye movement desensitization and reprocessing
EK400	Ektachem 400 (analysis for potassium, carbon dioxide, chloride, glucose, and blood urea nitrogen)		
		EMF	elective mid forceps
			endomyocardial fibrosis
			erythrocyte maturation factor
EKC	epidemic keratoconjuctivitis		

	evaporated milk formula	ENDO	endodontia
EMG	electromyograph		endodontics
	emergency		endoscopy
	essential monoclonal		endotracheal
	gammopathy	ENOG	electroneurography
EMIC	emergency maternity and	ENF	Enfamil®
	infant care	ENG	electronystagmogram
E-MICR	electron microscopy		engorged
EMIT	enzyme multiplied	ENL	erythema nodosum
	immunoassay technique		leprosum
EMLA®	eutectic mixture of local	ENP	extractable nucleoprotein
	anesthetics (lidocaine	ENT	ears, nose, throat
	and prilocaine in an	ENVD	elevated new vessels on
	emulsion base)		the disc
EMLB	erythromycin lactobionate	ENVE	elevated new vessels
EMMV	extended mandatory		elsewhere
	minute ventilation	ENVT	environment
EMR	educable mentally	EO	elbow orthosis
	retarded		eosinophilia
	electrical muscle		ethylene oxide
	stimulation		eyes open
	emergency mechanical	EOA	erosive osteoarthritis
	restraint		esophageal obturator
	empty, measure, and		airway
	record		examine, opinion, and
EMS	early morning stiffness		advice
	electrical muscle		external oblique
	stimulation		aponeurosis
	emergency medical	EOB	end of bed
	services	EOC	enema of choice
	eosinophilia myalgia	EOD	every other day (this is a
	syndrome		dangerous abbreviation)
EMT	emergency medical	EOG	electro-oculogram
	technician		Ethrane®, oxygen, and
EMTA	Emergency Medical		gas (nitrous oxide)
	Technician, Advanced	EOM	external otitis media
EMTP	Emergency Medical		extraocular movement
	Technician, Paramedic		extraocular muscles
EMV	eye, motor, verbal	EOMI	extraocular muscles intact
	(grading for Glasgow	EOR	emergency operating
	coma scale)		room
EMVC	early mitral valve closure	EORA	elderly onset rheumatoid
EMW	electromagnetic waves		arthritis
EN	enteral nutrition	eos.	eosinophil
	erythema nodosum	EP	ectopic pregnancy
ENA	extractable nuclear		electrophysiologic
	antigen		elopement precaution
ENB	esthesioneuroblastoma		endogenous pyrogen
ENC	encourage		Episcopal

	evoked potentials	EPT®	early pregnancy test
E&P	estrogen and progesterone	EPTS	existed prior to service
EPA	eicosapentaenoic acid	ER	emergency room
E-Panel	electrolyte panel (potassium, sodium, carbon dioxide, and chloride)		estrogen receptors external rotation
		E & R	equal and reactive examination and report
EPAP	expiratory positive airway pressure	ER+	estrogen receptor-positive
EPB	extensor pollicis brevis	ERA	estrogen receptor assay evoked response audiometry
EPC	erosive prephloric changes		
EPD	equilibrium peritoneal dialysis	ERCP	endoscopic retrograde cholangiopancreatography
EPEC	enteropathogen *Escherichia coli*	ERCT	emergency room computerized tomography
EPEG	etoposide		
EPF	Enfamil Premature Formula®	ERD	early retirement with disability
EPG	electronic pupillography	ERE	external rotation in extension
EPI	echo-planar imaging epinephrine epitheloid cells exocrine pancreatic insufficiency	ERF	external rotation in flexion
		ERFC	erythrocyte rosette forming cells
EPIS	episiotomy	ERG	electroretinogram
epith	epithelial	ERL	effective refractory length
EPL	extensor pollicis longus	ERNA	equilibrium radionuclide angiocardiography
EPM	electronic pacemaker		
EPO	epoetin alfa (erythropoietin) exclusive provider organization	ERP	effective refractory period emergency room physician endocardial resection procedure endoscopic retrograde pancreatography event-related potentials estrogen receptor protein
EPP	erythropoietic protoporphyria		
EPR	electrophrenic respiration emergency physical restraint estimated protein requirement		
		ERPF	effective renal plasma flow
EPS	electrophysiologic study extrapyramidal syndrome (symptom)	ER/PR	estrogen receptor/progesterone receptor
		ERS	endoscopic retrograde sphincterotomy
EPSDT	early periodic screening, diagnosis, and treatment	ERT	estrogen replacement therapy
EPSE	extrapyramidal side effects	ERV	expiratory reserve volume
EPSS	E point septal separation	ES	electrical stimulation emergency service

	end-to-side		ethionamide
	ex-smoker	*et al*	and others
	extra strength	ETC	and so forth
ESA	end-to-side anastomosis		estimated time of conception
ESAP	evoked sensory (nerve) action potential	ETCO₂	end tidal carbon dioxide
ESC	end systolic counts	ETD	eustachian tube dysfunction
ESD	Emergency Services Department	ETE	end-to-end
	esophagus, stomach, and duodenum	ETEC	enterotoxigenic *Escherichia coli*
ESF	external skeletal fixation	ETF	eustachian tubal function
ESLD	end-stage liver disease	ETH	elixir terpin hydrate
ESM	ejection systolic murmur		ethanol
	endolymphatic stromal myosis		Ethrane®
ESO	esophagus	ETHc̄C	elixir terpin hydrate with codeine
	esotropia	ETI	ejective time index
ESP	endometritis, salpingitis, and peritonitis	ETKTM	every test known to man
	end systolic pressure	ETO	estimated time of ovulation
	especially		ethylene oxide
	extrasensory perception		eustachian tube obstruction
ESR	erythrocyte sedimentation rate	ETOH	alcohol
ESRD	end-stage renal disease		alcoholic
ESRF	end-stage renal failure	ETOP	elective termination of pregnancy
ESS	emotional, spiritual, and social	ETP	elective termination of pregnancy
	essential	ETS	endotracheal suction
EST	electroshock therapy		end-to-side
	electrostimulation therapy		erythromycin topical solution
	exercise stress test	ETT	endotracheal tube
ESWL	extracorporeal shockwave lithotripsy		esophageal transit time
ET	ejection time		exercise tolerance test
	endotracheal		extrathyroidal thyroxine
	enterostomal therapy (therapist)	ETU	emergency and trauma unit
	esotropia		emergency treatment unit
	essential thrombocythemia	EU	equivalent units
	essential tremor		esophageal ulcer
	eustachian tube		etiology unknown
	exchange transfusion		excretory urography
	exercise treadmill	EUA	examine under anesthesia
ET′	esotropia for near	EUCD	emotionally unstable character disorder
et	and		
E(T)	intermittent esotropia	EUG	extrauterine gestation
ETA	endotracheal airway		

EUM	external urethral meatus	
EUP	extrauterine pregnancy	
EUS	external urethral sphincter	
EV	epidermodysplasia verruciformis	
	esophageal varices	
eV	electron volt (unit of radiation energy)	
EVA	ethylene vinyl acetate	
EVAC	evacuation	
eval	evaluate	
EVD	external ventricular drain	
EVE	evening	
EVS	endoscopic variceal sclerosis	
ew	elsewhere	
EWB	estrogen withdrawal bleeding	
EWCL	extended wear contact lens	
EWHO	elbow-wrist-hand orthosis	
EWL	estimated weight loss	
EWSCLs	extended-wear soft contact lenses	
EWT	erupted wisdom teeth	
ex	examined	
	excision	
	exercise	
exam.	examination	
EXEF	exercise ejection fraction	
EXH VT	exhaled tidal volume	
EXL	elixir	
EXOPH	exophthalmos	
EXP	experienced	
	exploration	
	expose	
expect	expectorant	
exp. lap.	exploratory laparotomy	
EXT	extension	
	external	
	extract	
	extraction	
	extremity	
Ext mon	external monitor	
extrav	extravasation	
ext. rot.	external rotation	
EXTUB	extubation	
EX U	excretory urogram	

F

F	facial
	Fahrenheit
	fair
	fasting
	father
	female
	finger
	firm
	flow
	fluoride
	French
	fundi
F/	full upper denture
/F	full lower denture
(F)	final
F_1	offspring from the first generation
F_2	offspring from the second generation
F II	factor II (two)
F VIII	factor VIII (8)
FA	femoral artery
	fluorescein angiogram
	folic acid
	forearm
FAA	febrile antigen agglutination
FAAP	family assessment adjustment pass
FAA SOL	formalin, acetic, and alcohol solution
FAAN	Fellow of the American Academy of Nursing
FAAP	Fellow of the American Academy of Pediatrics
FAB	digoxin immune Fab (Digibind®)
	French-American-British Cooperative group
	functional arm brace
FABER	full abduction and external rotation
FABF	femoral artery blood flow

63

FABM3	acute promyelocyte leukemia	FACOG	Fellow of the American College of Obstetricians & Gynecologists
FAC	fluorouracil, Adriamycin®, and cyclophosphamide		
		FACOS	Fellow of the American College of Orthopedic Surgeons
	fractional area concentration		
FACA	Fellow of the American College of Anaesthetists	FACP	Fellow of the American College of Physicians
		FACPRM	Fellow of the American College of Preventive Medicine
FACAG	Fellow of the American College of Angiology		
FACAL	Fellow of the American College of Allergists	FACR	Fellow of the American College of Radiology
FACAN	Fellow of the American College of Anesthesiologists	FACS	Fellow of the American College of Surgeons
			fluorescent-activated cell sorter
FACAS	Fellow of the American College of Abdominal Surgeons	FACSM	Fellow of the American College of Sports Medicine
FACC	Fellow of the American College of Cardiology	FAD	familial Alzheimer's disease
FACCP	Fellow of the American College of Chest Physicians		Family Assessment Device
			fetal abdominal diameter
FACCPC	Fellow of the American College of Clinical Pharmacology & Chemotherapy		flavin adenine dinucleotide
		FAE	fetal alcohol effect
		FAGA*	full-term appropriate for gestational age
FACD	Fellow of the American College of Dentists	FAI	Functional Assessment Inventory
FACEM	Fellow of the American College of Emergency Medicine	FALL	fallopian
		FAM	family
FACEP	Fellow of the American College of Emergency Physicians		fluorouracil, Adriamycin®, and mitomycin
FACGE	Fellow of the American College of Gastroenterology	FAMA	fluorescent antibody to membrane antigen
FACH	forceps to after-coming head	FAME	fluorouracil, doxorubicin, and methyl CCNU
FACLM	Fellow of the American College of Legal Medicine	FANA	fluorescent antinuclear antibody
		FAP	familial adenomatous polyposis
FACN	Fellow of the American College of Nutrition		familial amyloid polyneuropathy
FACNP	Fellow of the American College of Neuro-psychopharmacology		femoral artery pressure
			fibrillating action potential

F-ara-A	fludarabine phosphate	F. cath.	Foley catheter
FAS	fetal alcohol syndrome	FCBD	fibrocystic breast disease
FASHP	Fellow of the American Society of Hospital Pharmacists	FCC	familial colonic cancer family centered care femoral cerebral catheter follicular center cells fracture compound comminuted
FAST	fluorescent allergosorbent technique		
FAT	Fetal Activity Test fluorescent antibody test	FCCL	follicular center cell lymphoma
FAZ	foveal avascular zone	FCCU	family centered care unit
FB	fasting blood (sugar) finger breadth foreign body	FCD	fibrocystic disease
		FCDB	fibrocystic disease of the breast
F/B	followed by forward bending	FCE	fluorouracil, cisplatin, and etoposide
FBC	full blood count		
FBD	fibrocystic breast disease functional bowel disease	FCH	familial combined hyperlipidemia
FBF	forearm blood flow	FCHL	familial combined hyperlipemia
FBG	foreign-body-type granulomata	FCL	fibular collateral ligament
FBH	hydroxybutyric dehydrogenase	F-CL	fluorouracil and calcium leucovorin
FBI	full bony impaction	FCMC	family centered maternity care
FBL	fecal blood loss		
FBM	fetal breathing motion	FCMD	Fukiyama's congenital muscular dystrophy
FBRCM	fingerbreadth below right costal margin	FCMN	family centered maternity nursing
FBS	fasting blood sugar fetal bovine serum	FCP	formocresol pulpotomu
		FCR	flexor carpi radialis
FBU	fingers below umbilicus	FCRB	flexor carpi radialis brevis
FBW	fasting blood work	FCS	fever, chills, and sweating
FC	family conference febrile convulsion female child fever, chills financial class finger clubbing finger counting flexion contractor flucytosine Foley catheter foster care functional capacity functional class		
		FCSNVD	fever, chills, sweating, nausea, vomiting, and diarrhea
		FCU	flexor carpi ulnaris
		FD	familial dysautonomia fetal demise focal distance forceps delivery free drain full denture
5FC	flucytosine (this is a dangerous abbreviation as it can look like 5FU)		
		F & D	fixed and dilated
		FDA	Food and Drug Administration fronto-dextra anterior
F + C	flare and cells		
F & C	foam and condom	FDBL	fecal daily blood loss
		FDE	fixed drug eruption

FDG	feeding		sinus surgery
	fluorine-18-labeled deoxyglucose	FETI	fluorescence (fluorescent) energy transfer immunoassay
FDGS	feedings		
FDIU	fetal death in utero	FEUO	for external use only
FDLMP	first day of last menstrual period	FEV_1	forced expiratory volume in one second
FDM	fetus of diabetic mother flexor digiti minimi	$FEV_{1\%VC}$	forced expiratory volume in one second as percent of forced vital capacity
FDP	fibrin-degradation products		
	flexor digitorum profundus	FF	fat free fecal frequency filtration fraction
FDS	flexor digitorum superficialis for duration of stay		finger to finger flat feet force fluids foster father
Fe	female iron		fundus firm further flexion
FEC	fluorouracil, etoposide, and cisplatin	F&F	fixes and follows
	forced expiratory capacity	FF1/U	fundus firm 1 cm above umbilicus
FECG	fetal electrocardiogram	FF2/U	fundus firm 2 cm above umbilicus
FEF	forced expiratory flow rate	FF@u	fundus firm at umbilicus
$FEF_{25\%-75\%}$	forced expiratory flow during the middle half of the forced vital capacity	FFA	free fatty acid
		FFAT	Free Floating Anxiety Test
FEF_{x-y}	forced expiratory flow between two designated volume points in the forced vital capacity	FFB	flexible fiberoptic bronchoscopy
		FFD	fat-free diet focal-film distance
FEL	familial erythrophagocytic lymphohistiocytosis	FFI	fast food intake
FeLV	feline leukemia virus	FFM	fat-free mass five finger movement
FEM	femoral		
fem-fem	femoral-femoral (bypass)	FFP	fresh frozen plasma
Fem-pop	femoral popliteal (bypass)	FFS	fee-for-service
FEN	fluid, electrolytes, and nutrition		Fight For Sight flexible fiberoptic sigmoidoscopy
FENa	fractional extraction of sodium	FFT	fast-Fourier transforms flicker fusion threshold
FEP	free erythrocyte protoporphorin	FFTP	first full-term pregnancy
FES	fat embolism syndrome functional electrical stimulation	FFU/1	fundus firm 1 cm below umbilicus
		FFU/2	fundus firm 2 cm below umbilicus
$FeSO_4$	ferrous sulfate		
FESS	functional endoscopic	FG	fibrin glue

FGC	full gold crown		state precision
FGF	fibroblast growth factor	FITC	fluorescein isothiocyanate
FGP	fundic gland polyps	FIVC	forced inspiratory vital
FGS	focal segmental		capacity
	glomerulosclerosis	FJROM	full joint range of motion
FH	family history	FJS	finger joint size
	familial hypercholester-	FKE	full knee extension
	olemia	FL	fatty liver
	fetal head		fetal length
	fetal heart		fluid
	fundal height		flutamide and leuprolide
FHC	familial hypertrophic		acetate
	cardiomyopathy		full liquids
	family health center	fL	femtoliter (10^{-15} liter)
FHF	fulminant hepatic failure	FLA	free-living amebic
FHH	familial hypocalciuric		(ameba)
	hypercalcemia	FLASH	fast low-angle shot
	fetal heart heard	FLD	fatty liver disease
FHI	Fuch's heterochromic		fluid
	iridocyclitis		flutamide and leuprolide
FHL	flexor hallucis longus		acetate depot
FHNH	fetal heart not heard	FL Dtr	full lower denture
FHP	family history positive	flexsig	flexible sigmoidoscopy
FHR	fetal heart rate	FLGA	full-term, large for
FHRV	fetal heart rate variability		gestational age
FHS	fetal heart sounds	FLIC	Functional Living Index–
	fetal hydantoin syndrome		Cancer
FHT	fetal heart tone	FLK	funny looking kid (should
FIAC	fiacitabine		never be used: unusual
FIAU	fialuridine		facial features, is a
FiCO$_2$	fraction of inspired		better expression)
	carbon dioxide	fl. oz.	fluid ounce
FID	father in delivery	FL REST	fluid restriction
FIF	forced inspiratory flow	FLS	flashing lights and/ or
FIGLU	formiminoglutamic acid		scotoma
FIGO	International Federation	FLT	fluorothymidine
	of Gynecology and	FLU	fluconazole
	Obstetrics	FLU A	influenza A virus
FIL	father-in-law	FLW	fasting laboratory work
FIM	functional independence	FLZ	flurazepam
	measure	FM	face mask
FIND	follow-up intervention for		fat mass
	normal development		fetal movements
FiO$_2$	fraction of inspired	F & M	firm and midline (uterus)
	oxygen	FMC	fetal movement count
FIPT	periarteriolar transudate	FMD	family medical doctor
FISH	fluorescent in situ		fibromuscular dysplasia
	hybridization		foot and mouth disease
FISP	fast imaging with steady	FME	full mouth extraction

FMF	familial Mediterranean fever	FOB	father of baby
	fetal movement felt		fecal occult blood
	forced midexpiratory flow		feet out of bed
FMG	fine mesh gauze		fiberoptic bronchoscope
	foreign medical graduate		foot of bed
FMH	family medical history	FOBT	fecal occult blood test
	fibromuscular hyperplasia	FOC	father of child
FML®	fluorometholone		fluid of choice
FMN	first malignant neoplasm		fronto-occipital circumference
	flavin mononucleotide	FOD	fixing right eye
FMOL	femtomole		free of disease
FMP	fasting metabolic panel	FOEB	feet over edge of bed
	first menstrual period	FOG	Fluothane®, oxygen and gas (nitrous oxide)
FMPA	full mouth periapicals		
FMR	fetal movement record		full-on gain
FMRD	full mouth restorative dentistry	FOH	family ocular history
		FOI	flight of ideas
FMS	fluorouracil, mitomycin, and streptozocin	FOIA	Freedom of Information Act
	full mouth series	FOM	floor of mouth
FMV	fluorouracil, methyl-CCNU, and vincristine	FOMi	fluorouracil, Oncovin®, (vincristine), and mitomycin
FMX	full mouth x-ray	FOOB	fell out of bed
FN	false negative	FOOSH	fell on outstretched hand
	finger-to-nose	FOS	fiberoptic sigmoidoscopy
F/N	fluids and nutrition		fixing left eye
F to N	finger to nose	FOV	field of view
FNA	fine-needle aspiration	FOW	fenestration of oval window
FNAB	fine-needle aspiration biopsy		
		FP	false positive
FNAC	fine-needle aspiratory cytology		family planning
			family practice
FNCJ	fine needle catheter jejunostomy		family practitioner
			fibrous proliferation
FNF	finger nose finger		flat plate
FNH	focal nodular hyperplasia		food poisoning
FNR	false negative rate		frozen plasma
FNS	food and nutrition services	F-P	femoral popliteal
		fpA	fibrinopeptide A
	functional neuromuscular stimulation	F.P.A.L.	full term, premature, abortion, living
F/NS	fever and night sweats	FPB	femoral-popliteal bypass
FNT	finger to nose test		flexor pollicis brevis
FO	foot orthosis	FPC	familial polyposis coli
	foramen ovale		family practice center
	foreign object	FPD	feto-pelvic disproportion
	fronto-occipital		fixed partial denture

FPG	fasting plasma glucose
FPHx	family psychiatric history
FPIA	fluorescence-polarization immunoassay
FPL	flexor pollicis longus
FPM	full passive movements
FPNA	first-pass nuclear angiocardiography
FPU	family participation unit
FPZ	fluphenazine
FPZ-D	fluphenazine decanoate
FR	fair
	father
	Father (priest)
	flow rate
	fluid restriction
	Friends
F & R	force & rhythm (pulse)
FRA	fluorescent rabies antibody
FRACTS	fractional urines
FRC	frozen red cells
	functional residual capacity
FRE	flow-related enhancement
FREs	flow-related enhance-ments
FRF	filtration replacement fluid
FRJM	full range of joint movement
FROA	full range of affect
FROM	full range of motion
FS	fetoscope
	fingerstick
	flexible sigmoidoscopy
	fractional shortenings
	frozen section
	full strength
	functional status
F & S	full and soft
FSALO	Fletcher suite after loading ovoids
FSALT	Fletcher suite after loading tandem
FSB	fetal scalp blood
	full spine board
FSBM	full strength breast milk
FSC	flexible sigmoidoscopy

	fracture, simple and complete
FSD	focal-skin distance
	fracture, simple and depressed
FSE	fetal scalp electrode
FSG	focal and segmental glomerulosclerosis
FSGA	full-term, small for gestational age
FSGS	focal segmental glomerulosclerosis
FSH	facioscapulohumeral
	follicle stimulating hormone
FSHMD	facioscapulohumeral muscular dystrophy
FSIQ	Full-Scale Intelligence Quotient (part of Wechsler test)
FSM	functional status measures
F-SM/C	fungus, smear and culture
FSP	fibrin split products
FSS	fetal scalp sampling
	French steel sound (dilated to #24FSS)
	frequency-selective saturation
	full scale score
FSW	field service worker
FT	family therapy
	feeding tube
	filling time
	finger tip
	flexor tendon
	follow through
	foot (ft)
	full term
F_3T	trifluridine
FT_3	free triiodothyronine
FT_4	free thyroxine
FT_4I	free thyroxine index
FTA	fluorescent titer antibody
	fluorescent treponemal antibody
FTB	fingertip blood
FTBD	full-term born dead
FTC	full to confrontation
FTD	failure to descend

FTE	full-time equivalent	FUO	fever of undetermined origin
FTFTN	finger-to-finger-to-nose		
FTG	full thickness graft	FUOV	follow-up office visit
FTI	free thyroxine index	FU/LP	full upper denture, partial lower denture
FTKA	failed to keep appointment		
		FUS	fusion
FTLB	full-term living birth	FV	femoral vein
FTLFC	full-term living female child	FVC	false vocal cord(s)
			filled voiding flow rate
FTLMC	full-term living male child		forced vital capacity
FTM	fluid thioglycollate medium	FVH	focal vascular headache
		FVL	femoral vein ligation
FTN	finger-to-nose		flow volume loop
	full-term nursery	F waves	fibrillatory waves
FTNB	full-term newborn		flutter waves
FTND	full-term normal delivery	F/W	followed with
FTNSD	full-term, normal, spontaneous delivery	FWB	full weight bearing
		FWS	fetal warfarin syndrome
FTP	failure to progress	FWW	front wheel walker
FTR	father	Fx	fractional urine
	failed to report		fracture
	for the record	Fx-dis	fracture-dislocation
FTSD	full-term spontaneous delivery	FXN	function
		FXR	fracture
FTSG	full-thickness skin graft	FYC	facultative yeast carrier
FTT	failure to thrive	FYI	for your information
	fetal tissue transplant		
Ftube	feeding tube		
FTV	functional trial visit		
FU	fraction unbound		
F & U	flanks and upper quadrants		

G

F/U	follow-up	G	gallop
	fundus at umbilicus		gastrostomy
F↑U	fingers above umbilicus		gauge
F↓U	fingers below umbilicus		good
5-FU	fluorouracil		grade
FUB	function uterine bleeding		gram (g)
FUDR®	floxuridine		gravida
FU Dtr	full upper denture		guaiac
FUF		G +	gram-positive
FU/FL	full upper denture, full lower denture	G −	gram-negative
		G1–4	grade 1–4
FULG	fulguration	G-11	hexachlorophene
5FU/LV	fluorouracil and leucovorin	GA	Gamblers Anonymous
			gastric analysis
FUN	follow-up note		
FUNG-C	fungus culture		
FUNG-S	fungus smear		

	general anesthesia
	general appearance
	gestational age
	ginger ale
	granuloma annulare
	glucose/acetone
Ga	gallium
GABA	gamma-aminobutyric acid
GABHS	group A beta hemolytic streptococci
GAD	generalized anxiety disorder
GAG	glycosaminoglycan
Gal	gallon
G'ale	ginger ale
GALI-PUT	galactose-1-phosphate uridyle transferase enzyme
GAR	gonnococcal antibody reaction
GAS	general adaption syndrome
	Glasgow Assessment Schedule
	Global Assessment Scale
	group A streptococcus
Gas Anal F&T	gastric analysis, free and total
Ga scan	gallium scan
Gastroc	gastrocnemius
GAT	group adjustment therapy
GATB	General Aptitude Test Battery
GAU	geriatric assessment unit
Gaw	airway conductance
GB	gallbladder
	Guillain-Barré (syndrome)
G & B	good and bad
GBA	ganglionic-blocking agent
GBBS	group B beta hemolytic streptococcus
GBE	*Ginkgo biloba* extract
GBH	gamma benzene hexachloride (lindane)
GBM	glioblastoma multiforme
	glomerular basement membrane
GBMI	guilty but mentally ill
GBP	gated blood pool (imaging)

	gastric bypass
GBR	good blood return
GBS	gallbladder series
	gastric bypass surgery
	group B streptococci
	Guillain-Barré syndrome
GC	gas chromatography
	geriatric chair (Gerichair®)
	gonococci (gonorrhea)
	good condition
	graham crackers
GCI	General Cognitive Index
G−C	gram-negative cocci
G+C	gram-positive cocci
GCA	giant cell arteritis
GCE	general conditioning exercise
GCDFP	gross cystic disease fluid protein
GCIIS	glucose control insulin infusion system
GCL	good clinical practice (principles of)
GCM	good central maintained
GCS	Glasgow Coma Scale
G-CSF	filgrastim (granulocyte colony-stimulating factor)
GCST	Gibson-Cooke sweat test
GCT	general care and treatment
	germ cell tumor
	giant cell tumor
GCU	gonococcal urethritis
GD	gestational diabetes
	Graves' disease
Gd	gadolinium
G and D	growth and development
GDA	gastroduodenal artery
GDF	gel diffusion precipitin
GDM	gestational diabetes mellitus
GE	gainfully employed
	gastric emptying
	gastroenteritis
	gastroesophageal
GEC	galactose elimination capacity
GEE	Global Evaluation of Efficacy

GEN/ ENDO	general anesthesia with endotracheal intubation		gastrointestinal bleeding
		GIC	general immunocompetence
GENT	gentamicin		
GENTA/P	gentamicin-peak	GIDA	Gastrointestinal Diagnostic Area
GENTA/T	gentamicin-trough		
GEP	gastroenteropancreatic	GIFT	gamete intrafallopian transfer
GEQ	generic equiavalent		
GER	gastroesophageal reflux	GIK	glucose-insulin-potassium
GERD	gastroesophageal reflux disease	GILO	glioblastoma
		ging	gingiva
GET	gastric emptying time	GIP	gastric inhibitory peptide
	graded exercise test		giant cell interstitial pneumonia
GETA	general endotracheal anesthesia		
		GIS	gas in stomach
GF	gastric fistula		gastrointestinal series
	gluten free	GIT	gastrointestinal tract
	grandfather	GITS	gastrointestinal therapeutic system
GFAP	glial fibrillary acid protein		
GFCL	Goldmann fundus contact lens	GITSG	Gastrointestinal Tumor Study Group
		GITT	glucose insulin tolerance test
GFD	gluten-free diet		
GFM	good fetal movement	GIWU	gastrointestinal work-up
GFR	glomerular filtration rate	giv	given
	grunting, flaring, and retractions	GJ	gastrojejunostomy
		GL	gastric lavage
GFS	glaucoma filtering surgery		glaucoma
GG	gamma globulin		greatest length
	guaifenesin	GLA	gingivolinguoaxial
G=G	grips equal and good	GLC	gas-liquid chromatography
GGE	generalized glandular enlargement		
		GLP	Gambro Liendia Plate
GGS	glands, goiter, and stiffness		good laboratory practice (principles of)
GGT	gamma-glutamyl transferase	GLR	gravity lumbar reduction
		GLU 5	five hour glucose tolerance test
GGTP	gamma-glutamyl transpeptidase		
GH	growth hormone	GLYCOS Hb	glycosylated hemoglobin
GHB	gamma hydroxybutyrate		
GHb	glycosylated hemoglobin	GM	gram
GHD	growth hormone deficiency		grand mal
			grandmother
G-Hjt	glenohumeral joint	GM +	gram-positive
GHP(S)	gated heart pool (scan)	GM –	gram-negative
GHQ	General Health Questionnaire	gm %	grams per 100 milliliters
		GMC	general medical clinic
GI	gastrointestinal	GM-CSF	sargramostim (granulocyte-macrophage
	granuloma inguinale		
GIB	gastric ileal bypass		

72

	colony-stimulating factor)		grandparent
GMF	general medical floor		gutta percha
GMH	germinal matrix hemorrhage	G/P	gravida/para
		G_4P_{3104}	four pregnancies (gravid), 3 went to term, one premature, no abortion (or miscarriage), and 4 living children (p = para)
GMP	guanosine monophosphate		
GMS	general medical services		
	general medicine and surgery		
	Gomori methenamine silver	GPC	giant papillary conjunctivitis
GM&S	general medicine and surgery		gram-positive cocci
GMTs	geometric mean antibody titers	GPC/TP	glycerylphosphorylcholine to total phosphate
GN	glomerulonephritis	G6PD	glucose-6-phosphate dehydrogenase
	graduate nurse		
	gram-negative	G-PLT	giant platelets
GNB	gram-negative bacilli	GPMAL	gravida, para, multiple births, abortions, and live births
	gram-negative bacteremia		
GND	gram-negative diplococci		
GNID	gram-negative intracellular diplococci	GPN	graduate practical nurse
		GPS	Goodpasture's syndrome
GNR	gram-negative rods	GPT	glutamic pyruvic transaminase
GnRH	gonadotropin-releasing hormone	gr	grain (approximately 60 mg) (this is a dangerous abbreviation)
GNS	gram-negative sepsis		
GnSAF	gonadotropin surge attenuating factor	G−R	gram-negative rods
		G+R	gram-positive rods
GOCS	Global Obsessive-Compulsive Scale	GRASS	gradient recalled acquisition in a steady state
GOD	glucose oxidase		
GOG	Gynecologic Oncology Group	Grav.	gravid (pregnant)
		GRD	gastroesophageal reflux disease
GOK	God only knows		
GOMER	get out of my emergency room	GRE	graded resistive exercise
			gradient refocused echo
GON	gonococcal ophthalmia neonatorum	GR-FR	grandfather
		GR-MO	grandmother
	greater occipital neuritis	GRN	granules
GOO	gastric outlet obstruction		green
GOR	general operating room	GRP	group
GOT	glucose oxidase test	$Gr_1P_0AB_1$	one pregnancy, no births, and one abortion
	glutamic-oxaloacetic transaminase (aspartate aminotransferase)		
		GRT	gastric residence time
	goals of treatment		Graduate Respiratory Therapist
GP	general practitioner		
	glucose polymers	GRTT	Graduate Respiratory Therapist Technician
	gram-positive		

GS	gallstone	GTT agar	gelatin-tellurite-taurocholate agar
	generalized seizure	GTT3H	glucose tolerance test 3 hours (oral)
	general surgery		
	Gram stain	GTTS	drops
	grip strength	GU	genitourinary
G/S	5% dextrose (glucose) and 0.9% sodium chloride (saline) injection	GUAR	guarantor
		GUS	genitourinary sphincter genitourinary system
GSD	glucogen storage disease	GUSTO	Global Utilization of Streptokinase and TPA for Occluded Coronary Arteries
GSD-1	glycogen storage disease, type 1		
GSE	genital self-examination		
	gluten sensitive enteropathy	GVF	Goldmann visual fields good visual fields
	grip strong and equal	GVHD	graft-versus-host disease
GSI	genuine stress incontinence	GVN	gentamicin, vancomycin, and nystatin
GSP	general survey panel	G/W	glucose water
GSPN	greater superficial petrosal neurectomy	G&W	glycerin and water (enema)
GSR	galvanic skin resistance (response)	GWA	gunshot wound of the abdomen
	gastrosalivary reflex	GWT	gunshot wound of the throat
GST	gold sodium thiomalate		
GSTM	gold sodium thiomalate	GXP	graded exercise program
GSW	gunshot wound	GZTS	Guilford-Zimmerman Temperament Survey
GSWA	gunshot wound to abdomen		
GT	gait		
	gait training		
	gastrotomy tube		
	group therapy		**H**
GTC	generalized tonic-clonic (seizure)		
GTCS	generalized tonic-clonic seizure		
GTD	gestational trophoblastic disease	H	*Haemophilis*
			heart
GTF	gastrostomy tube feedings		height
	glucose tolerence factor		heroin
GTN	gestational trophoblastic neoplasms		Hispanic
			hour
	glomerulo-tubulo-nephritis		husband
GTP	glutamyl transpeptidase		hydrogen
GTS	Gilles de la Tourette syndrome		hyperopia
			hypermetropia
GTT	drop		hypodermic
	glucose tolerance test	Ⓗ	hypodermic injection

H²	hiatal hernia	HAP	hearing aid problem
H₂	hydrogen		hospital-acquired
3H	high, hot, and a helluva		pneumonia
	lot	HAPC	hospital-acquired
HA	headache		penetration contact
	hearing aid	HAPE	high altitude pulmonary
	heart attack		edema
	hemadsorption	HAPS	hepatic arterial perfusion
	hemolytic anemia		scintigraphy
	hospital admission	HAPTO	haptoglobin
	hyperalimentation	HAQ	Headache Assessment
	hypermetropic		Questionnaire
	astigmatism		Health Assessment
	hypothalmic amenorrhea		Questionnaire
H/A	head-to-abdomen (ratio)	HAR	high altitude retinopathy
HA-1A®	nebacumab	HARH	high altitude retinal
HAA	hepatitis-associated		hemorrhage
	antigen	HARS	Hamilton Anxiety Rating
HAAB	hepatitis A antibody		Scale
HACS	hyperactive child	HAS	Hamilton Anxiety
	syndrome		(Rating) Scale
HAD	human adjuvant disease		hyperalimentation solution
HAE	hearing aid evaluation	HASHD	hypertensive
	hepatic artery		arteriosclerotic heart
	embolization		disease
	hereditary angioedema	HAT	head, arms, and trunk
HAF	hyperalimentation fluid		hospital arrival time
HAGG	hyperimmune antivariola	HAV	hallux abducto valgus
	gamma globulin		hepatitis A virus
HAI	hemagglutination	HB	heart block
	inhibition assay		heel to buttock
	hepatic arterial infusion		hemoglobin (Hb)
HAL	hyperalimentation		hold breakfast
HALO	halothane		housebound
HAM	HTLV-1-associated	1⁰HB	first degree heart block
	myelopathy	HBAB	hepatitis B antibody
	human albumin	HbA₁c	glycosylated hemoglobin
	microspheres	HBAC	hyperdynamic
HAMA	human anti-murine		beta-adrenergic
	antibody		circulatory
HAM-A	Hamilton Anxiety (scale)	HbAS	sickle cell trait
HAM D	Hamilton Depression	HBBW	hold breakfast for blood
	(scale)		work
HAMS	hamstrings	HBcAb	hepatitis B core antibody
HAN	heroin associated		(antigen)
	nephropathy	HBc AB	hepatitis B core antibody
HANE	hereditary angioneurotic	HBc AG	hepatitis B core antigen
	edema	HB core	hepatits B core antigen
HAO	hearing aid orientation	HBD	has been drinking

	hydroxybutyric acid dehydrogenase		housecall
HBF	fetal hemoglobin		hydrocephalus
	hepatic blood flow		hydrocortisone
HBGA	had it before, got it again	H & C	hot and cold
HBGM	home blood glucose monitoring	HCA	health care aide
HBH	Health Belief Model	H-CAP	hexamethylmelamine, cyclophosphamide, doxorubicin, and cisplatin
HBI	hemibody irradiation		
HBID	hereditary benign intraepithelial dyskeratosis	HCC	hepatocellular carcinoma
		HCD	hydrocolloid dressing
HBIG	hepatitis B immune globulin	HCFA	Health Care Financing Administration
Hb Kansas	mutant hemoglobin with a low affinity for oxygen	HCG	human chorionic gonadotropin
HBLV	B-lymphotropic virus human	HCH	hexachlorocyclohexane
		HCl	hydrochloric acid
HBO	hyperbaric oxygen		hydrochloride
HbO_2	hyperbaric oxygen	HCL	hairy cell leukemia
	hemoglobin, oxygenated	HCLs	hard contact lenses
HBOT	hyperbaric oxygen treatment	HCLV	hairy cell leukemia variant
HBP	high blood pressure	HCM	health care maintenance
HBPM	home blood pressure monitoring		hypercalcemia of malignancy
			hypertropic cardiomyopa-thy
HBS	Health Behavior Scale		
HbS	sickle cell hemoglobin	HCMV	human cytomegalovirus infections
HBsAg	hepatitis B surface antigen	HCO_3	bicarbonate
HbSC	sickle cell hemoglobin C	HCP	hereditary coporphyria
HBSS	Hank's balanced salt solution	HCS	human chorionic somatomammotropin
HbSS	sickle cell anemia	17-HCS	17-hydroxycorticosteroids
HBT	hydrogen breath test	HCT	head computerized (axial) tomography
HBV	hepatitis B vaccine		hematocrit
	hepatitis B virus		histamine challenge test
	honey-bee venom		human chorionic thyrotropin
HBVP	high biological value protein		hydrochlorothiazide (this is a dangerous abbreviation)
HBW	high birth weight		
H/BW	heart-to-body weight (ratio)		hydrocortisone
HC	handicapped	HCTU	home cervical traction unit
	head circumference	HCTZ	hydrochlorothiazide (this is a dangerous abbreviation)
	heel cords		
	Hickman catheter		
	home care		
	hot compress		

HCV	hepatitis C virus
HCVD	hypertensive cardiovascular disease
HCWs	health-care workers
HD	haloperidol decanoate
	hearing distance
	heart disease
	heloma durum
	hemodialysis
	high dose
	hip disarticulation
	Hodgkin's disease
	hospital day
	hospital discharge
	house dust
	Huntington's disease
HDAC	high-dose cytarabine
HDARAC	high-dose cytarabine (ARA C)
HDCV	rabies virus vaccine, human diploid (human diploid cell vaccine)
HDH	high-density humidity
HDL	high-density lipoprotein
HDLW	hearing distance for watch in left ear
HDMTX	high-dose methotrexate
HDMTX-CF	high-dose methotrexate and citrovorum factor
HDMTX/LV	high-dose methotrexate and leucovorin
HDN	hemolytic disease of the newborn
	high-density nebulizer
HDP	high-density polyethylene
	hydroxymethyline diphosphonate
HDPAA	heparin-dependent platelet-associated antibody
HDRS	Hamilton Depression Rating Scale
HDRW	hearing distance for watch in right ear
HDS	Hamilton Depression (Rating) Scale
HDU	hemodialysis unit
HDV	hepatitis delta virus
HE	hard exudate

H&E	hematoxylin and eosin
	hemorrhage and exudate
	heredity and environment
HEA	health
HEAT	human erythrocyte agglutination test
HEC	Health Education Center
HEENT	head, eyes, ears, nose, and throat
HEK	human embryonic kidney
HEL	human embryonic lung
HELA	Helen Lake (tumor cells)
HELLP Syndrome	hemolysis, elevated liver enzymes, and low platelet count
HEMA	hydroxyethylmethacrylate
HEMI	hemiplegia
HEMOSID	hemosiderin
HEMPAS	hereditary erythrocytic multinuclearity with positive acidified serum test
HEMS	helicopter emergency medical services
HEP	heparin
	hepatic
	histamine equivalent prick
	home exercise program
HEPA	hamster egg penetration assay
hep cap	heparin cap
HERP	human exposure (dose)/rodent potency (dose)
HES	hydroxyethyl starch (hetastarch)
	hypereosinophilic syndrome
HEV	hepato-encephalomyelitis virus
Hex	hexamethylmelamine
Hexa-CAF	hexamethylmelamine, cyclophosphamide, methotrexate, and fluorouracil
HF	hard feces
	hay fever
	head of fetus
	heart failure

	high frequency	HHNC	hyperosmolar hyperglycemic nonketotic coma
	Hispanic female		
	hot flashes		
	house formula	HHNK	hyperglycemic hyperosmolar nonketotic (coma)
HFA	health facility administrator		
HFD	high fiber diet	HHS	Health and Human Service (US Department of)
	high forceps delivery		
HFHL	high-frequence hearing loss	HHT	hereditary hemorrhagic telangiectasis
HFI	hereditary fructose intolerance	HHTC	high-humidity trach collar
HFJV	high frequency jet ventilation	HHTM	high-humidity trach mask
H flu	*Haemophilus influenzae*	HHTS	high-humidity tracheostomy shield
HFO	high-frequency oscillation	HI	head injury
HFPPV	high-frequency positive pressure ventilation		hearing impaired
			hemagglutination inhibition
HFST	hearing-for-speech test		hospital insurance
HFUPR	hourly fetal urine production rate	HIA	hemagglutination inhibition antibody
HFV	high-frequency ventilation	HIAA	hydroxyindoleacetic acid
HG	hemoglobin	5-HIAA	5-hydroxyindoleacetic acid
Hgb	hemoglobin		
HGH	human growth hormone	HIB	*Haemophilus influenzae* type b (vaccine)
HGO	hip guidance orthosis		
HGPRT	hypoxanthine-guanine phosphoribosyl-transferase	hi-cal	high caloric
		HID	headache, insomnia, and depression
HH	hard of hearing		
	hiatal hernia		herniated intervertebral disc
	home health		
	household	HIDA	hepato-iminodiacetic acid (lidofenin)
	hypogonadotropic hypogonadism	HIE	hyperimmunoglobuline-mia E
H&H	hematocrit and hemoglobin		hypoxic-ischemic encephalopathy
HHA	hereditary hemolytic anemia	HIF	*Haemophilus influenzae*
	home health agency		higher integrative functions
	home health aid		
HHC	home health care	HIHA	high impulsiveness, high anxiety
HHD	home hemodialysis	HIL	hypoxic-ischemic lesion
	hypertensive heart disease	HILA	high impulsiveness, low anxiety
HHFM	high-humidity face mask		
HHM	high-humidity mask	HINI	hypoxic-ischemic neuronal injury
	humoral hypercalcemia of malignancy	hi-pro	high protein
HHN	hand held nebulizer		

HIR	head injury routine	HLT	heart-lung transplantation (transplant)
HIS	Hanover Intensive Score		
	Health Intention Scale	HLV	herpes-like virus
	Home Incapacity Scale		hypoplastic left ventricle
	hospital information system	HM	hand motion
			heart murmur
HISMS	How I See Myself Scale		heavily muscled
Histo	histoplasmin skin test		hemola molle
HIT	heparin induced thrombocytopenia		Hispanic male
			Holter monitor
	histamine inhalation test		human milk
	home infusion therapy		human semisynthetic insulin
HIU	head injury unit		
HIV	human immunodeficiency virus		humidity mask
		HMA	hemorrhages and microaneurysms
HIVD	herniated intervertebral disc		
		HMB	homatropine methylbromide
hi-vit	high vitamin		
HIVMP	high-dose intravenous methylprednisolone	HMBA	hexamethylene bisacetamide
HJB	Howell-Jolly bodies	HMD	hyaline membrane disease
HJR	hepato-jugular reflux	HME	heat, massage, and exercise
H-K	hand to knee		
HKAFO	hip-knee-ankle-foot orthosis		home medical equipment
		HMDP	hydroxymethyline diphosphonate
HKAO	hip-knee-ankle orthosis		
HKO	hip-knee orthosis	HMETSC	heavy metal screen
HKS	heel, knee, and shin	HMG	human menopausal gonadotropin
HL	hairline		
	half-life	HMG CoA	hepatic hydroxymethyl glutaryl coenzyme A
	hallux limitus		
	haloperidol	HMI	healed myocardial infarction
	harelip		
	hearing level	HMK	homemaking
	hemilaryngectomy	HMM	altretamine (hexamethyl-melamine)
	heparin lock		
	Hickman line	HMO	Health Maintenance Organization
H&L	heart and lung		
HLA	human lymphocyte antigen	HMP	hexose monophosphate
			hot moist packs
HLA nega-tive	heart, lungs, and abdomen negative	HMPAO	hexamethylpropylenamine oxide
HLD	haloperidol decanoate	HMR	histocytic medullary reticulosis
	herniated lumbar disc		
HLH	hemophagocytic lymphohistiocytosis	HMS	hyperactive malarial splenomegaly
			hypodermic morphine sulfate (this is a dangerous abbreviation)
HLHS	hypoplastic left heart syndrome		
HLK	heart, liver, and kidney		

HMS®	medrysone	HOI	hospital onset of infection
HMSN I	hereditary motor and sensory neuropathy type I	HOM	high-osmolar contrast media
HMWK	high molecular weight kininogen	HONDA	hypertensive, obese, Negro, diabetic, arthritic
HMX	heat massage exercise	HONK	hyperosmolar nonketotic (coma)
HN	head and neck		
	head nurse	HOPI	history of present illness
	high nitrogen	HORF	high-output renal failure
H&N	head and neck	HP	hard palate
HN₂	mechlorethamine HCl		*Helicobacter pylori*
HNC	hyperosmolar nonketotic coma		hemipelvectomy
			hemiplegia
HNI	hospitalization not indicated		hot packs
			hydrogen peroxide
HNKDC	hyperosomolar nonketotic diabetic coma		hydrophilic petrolatum
		H&P	history and physical
HNKDS	hyperosmolar nonketotic diabetic state	HPA	hypothalamic-pituitary-adrenal (axis)
HNLN	hospitalization no longer necessary	HPCE	high performance capillary electrophoresis
HNP	herniated nucleus pulposus	HPE	history and physical examination
HNRNA	heterogeneous nuclear ribonucleic acid	HPF	high-power field
		HPFH	hereditary persistence of fetal hemoglobin
HNS	head and neck surgery		
	head, neck, and shaft	HPG	human pituitary gonadotropin
HNV	has not voided		
HO	hand orthosis	HPI	history of present illness
	Hemotology-Oncology	HPL	human placenta lactogen
	heterotropic ossification		hyperplexia
	hip orthosis	HPLC	high-pressure (performance) liquid chromatography
	house officer		
H/O	history of		
H₂O	water	HPM	hemiplegic migraine
H₂O₂	hydrogen peroxide	HPN	home parenteral nutrition
HOA	hip osteoarthritis	HPO	hydrophilic ointment
HOB	head of bed		hypertrophic pulmonary osteoarthropathy
HOB UPSOB	head of bed up for shortness of breath		
		HPOA	hypertrophic pulmonary osteoarthropathy
HOC	Health Officer Certificate		
HOCM	high-osmolality contrast media	2HPP	2-hour postprandial (blood sugar)
	hypertrophic obstructive cardiomyopathy	2HPPBS	2-hour postprandial blood sugar
HOG	halothane, oxygen, and gas (nitrous oxide)	HPS	hypertrophic pyloric stenosis
HOH	hard of hearing		

HPT	histamine provocation test	
	hyperparathyroidism	
hPTH	human parathyroid hormone I$_{34}$ (teriparatide)	
HPTM	home prothrombin time monitoring	
HPV	human papilloma virus	
	human parvovirus	
HPZ	high pressure zone	
HQC	hydroquinone cream	
HR	hallux rigidus	
	Harrington rod	
	heart rate	
	hemorrhagic retinopathy	
	hospital record	
	hour	
H & R	hysterectomy and radiation	
HRA	high right atrium	
	histamine releasing activity	
H2RA	H2-receptor antagonist	
HRC	Human Rights Committee	
HRCT	high-resolution computed tomography	
HRF	Harris return flow	
	health-related facility	
	histamine releasing factor	
HRIF	histamine inhibitory releasing factor	
HRL	head rotated left	
HRLA	human reovirus-like agent	
HRLM	high-resolution light microscopy	
hRLX-2	synthetic human relaxin	
HRP	high-risk pregnancy	
	horseradish peroxidase	
HRR	head rotated right	
HRS	hepatorenal syndrome	
HRSD	Hamilton Rating Scale for Depression	
HRT	heart rate	
	heparin response test	
	hormone replacement therapy	
HS	bedtime	
	half strength	
	hamstrings	

	Hartman's solution (lactated Ringer's)	
	heart sounds	
	heavy smoker	
	heel spur	
	heel stick	
	hereditary spherocytosis	
	herpes simplex	
	high school	
H→S	heel to shin	
H&S	hemorrhage and shock	
	hysterectomy and sterilization	
HSA	Health Systems Agency	
	human serum albumin	
	hypersomnia-sleep apnea	
HSB	husband	
HSBG	heel stick blood gas	
HSCL	Hopkins Symptom Check List	
HSE	herpes simplex encephalitis	
HSG	herpes simplex genitalis	
	histosalpingogram	
HSK	herpes simplex keratitis	
HSL	herpes simplex labialis	
HSM	hepatosplenomegaly	
	holosystolic murmur	
HSN	Hansen-Street nail	
	heart sounds normal	
HSP	Henoch-Schönlein purpura	
	hysterosalpingography	
HSQ	Health Status Questionnaire	
HSR	heated serum reagin	
HSSE	high soap suds enema	
HSV	herpes simplex virus	
HSVI	herpes simplex virus type 1	
HSV2	herpes simplex virus type 2	
HT	hammertoe	
	hearing test	
	heart	
	heart transplant	
	height	
	high temperature	
	hyperthermia	

	Hubbard tank	HUS	hemolytic uremic syndrome
	hypermetropia		husband
	hyperopia	husb	husband
	hypertension	HV	hallux valgus
H&T	hospitalization and treatment		has voided
H(T)	intermittent hypertropia		Hemovac®
5-HT	serotonin (5-hydroxytryptamine)		home visit
ht. aer.	heated aerosol	H&V	hemigastrecotomy and vagotomy
HTAT	human tetanus antitoxin	HVA	homovanillic acid
HTB	hot tub bath	HVD	hypertensive vascular disease
HTC	heated tracheostomy collar	HVES	high voltage electrical stimulation
	hypertensive crisis	HVGS	high volt galvanic stimulation
HTF	house tube feeding		
HTK	heel to knee	HVL	half value layer
HTL	hearing threshold level	HW	heparin well
	human T-cell leukemia		homework
	human thymic leukemia		housewife
HTLV III	human T-cell lymphotrophic virus type III	hwb	hot water bottle
		HWFE	housewife
HTM	high threshold mechanoceptors	HWP	hot wet pack
		Hx	history
HTN	hypertension		hospitalization
HTO	high tibia osteotomy	HXM	hexamethylmelamine
HTP	House-Tree-Person-test	Hx & Px	history and physical (examination)
5-HTP	serotonin (5-hydroxytryptophan)		
		Hy	hypermetropia
HTS	head traumatic syndrome	HYDRO	hydronephrosis
	heel-to-shin	HYG	hygiene
	Hematest® stools	Hyper Al	hyperalimentation
HTSCA	human tumor stem cell assay	Hyper K	hyperkalemia
		Hypo K	hypokalemia
HTT	hand thrust test	hypopit	hypopituitarism
HTV	herpes-type virus	Hyst	hysterectomy
HTVD	hypertensive vascular disease	Hz	Hertz
		HZ	herpes zoster
HTX	hemothorax	HZO	herpes zoster ophthalmicus
HU	head unit		
	hydroxyurea	HZV	herpes zoster virus
Hu	Hounsfield units		
HUF	Humphrey's visual fields		
HUH	Humana Hospital		
HUIFM	human leukocyte interferon meloy		**I**
HUK	human urinary kallikrein	I	impression
HUR	hydroxyurea		incisal

	independent	IAV	intermittent assist ventilation
	initial		
	inspiration	IB	ileal bypass
	intact (bag of waters)		isolation bed
	intermediate	IBBB	intra-blood-brain barrier
	iris	IBBBB	incomplete bilateral bundle branch block
	one		
I_2	iodine	IBC	iron binding capacity
I^{131}	radioactive iodine	IBD	inflammatory bowel disease
IA	incidental appendectomy		
	intra-amniotic	IBDQ	Inflammatory Bowel Disease Questionnaire
I & A	irrigation and aspiration		
IAA	interrupted aortic arch	IBG	iliac bone graft
IAB	induced abortion	IBI	intermittent bladder irrigation
IABC	intra-aortic balloon counterpulsation		
		ibid	at the same place
IABP	intra-aortic balloon pump	IBILI	indirect bilirubin
IAC	internal auditory canal	IBNR	incurred but not reported
	intra-arterial chemotherapy	IBOW	intact bag of waters
		IBPS	Insall-Burstein posterior stabilizer
IAC-CPR	interposed abdominal compressions—cardiopulmonary resuscitation		
		IBRS	Inpatient Behavior Rating Scale
IACG	intermittent angle-closure glaucoma	IBS	irritable bowel syndrome
		IBU	ibuprofen
IACP	intra-aortic counterpulsation	IBW	ideal body weight
		IC	between meals
IADHS	inappropriate antidiuretic hormone syndrome		immunocompromised
			incomplete
IA DSA	intra-arterial subtraction arteriography		indirect Coombs (test)
			individual counseling
IAGT	indirect antiglobulin test		inspiratory capacity
IAHA	immune adherence hemagglutination		intensive care
			intercostal
IAI	intra-abdominal infection		intercourse
	intra-amniotic infection		intermediate care
IAM	internal auditory meatus		intermittent catheterization
IAN	intern's admission note		
IAO	immediately after onset		interstitial changes
IAP	intermittent acute porphyria		interstitial cystitis
			intracoronary
IART	intra-atrial reentrant tachycardia		intracranial
			intraincisional
IAS	idiopathic ankylosing spondylitis		irritable colon
		ICA	intermediate care area
IASD	interatrial septal defect		internal carotid artery
	immunoaugmentive therapy		islet-cell antibody
		ICAM	intracellular adhesion molecule
IAT	indirect antiglobulin test		

ICAT	infant cardiac arrest tray	ICR	intercostal retractions
ICB	intracranial bleeding	ICRF-159	razoxane
ICBG	iliac crest bone graft	ICS	ileocecal sphincter
ICBT	intercostobronchial trunk		intercostal space
ICC	islet cell carcinoma	ICSH	interstitial cell-stimulating hormone
ICCE	intracapsular cataract extraction	ICSR	intercostal space retractions
ICCU	intensive coronary care unit	ICT	icterus
	intermediate coronary care unit		indirect Coombs' test
			inflammation of connective tissue
ICD	instantaneous cardiac death		intensive conventional therapy
	isocitrate dehydrogenase		intermittent cervical traction
	irritant contact dermatitis		intracranial tumor
ICDC	implantable cardioverter-defibrillator catheter		islet cell transplant
		ICTX	intermittent cervical traction
ICD 9 CM	International Classification of Diseases, 9th Revision, Clinical Modification	ICU	intensive care unit
			intermediate care unit
ICDO	international classification of diseases for oncology	ICV	intracerebroventricular
		ICVH	ischemic cerebrovascular headache
ICE	ice, compression, and elevation	ICW	intercellular water
		ID	identification
	ifosfamide, carboplatin, and etoposide		identify
			ifosfamide, mesna uroprotection, and doxorubicin
	individual career exploration		
ICF	intermediate care facility		immunodiffusion
	intracellular fluid		infectious disease (physician or department)
ICG	indocyanine green		
ICH	immunocompromised host		initial diagnosis
	intracerebral hemorrhage		initial dose
	intracranial hemorrhage		intradermal
ICIT	intensified conventional insulin therapy	*id*	the same
ICL	intracorneal lens	I & D	incision and drainage
ICLE	intracapsular lens extraction	IDA	iron deficiency anemia
		IDC	idiopathic dilated cardiomyopathy
ICM	intracostal margin		
ICN	infection control nurse	IDDM	insulin-dependent diabetes mellitus
	intensive care nursery		
ICN2	neonatal intensive care unit level II	IDDS	implantable drug delivery system
ICP	intracranial pressure	IDE	Investigational Device Exemption
ICPP	intubated continuous positive pressure		

IDFC	immature dead female child		intrinsic factor
IDG	interdisciplinary group		involved field (radiotherapy)
IDI	Interpersonal Dependency Inventory	IFA	indirect fluorescent antibody immunofluorescent assay
IDK	internal derangement of knee	IFE	immunofixation electrophoresis
IDL	intermediate-density lipoprotein	IFM	internal fetal monitoring
IDM	infant of a diabetic mother	IFN	interferon
		IFOS	ifosfamide
IDMC	immature dead male child	IFP	inflammatory fibroid polyps
IDPN	intradialytic parenteral nutrition	IFSE	internal fetal scalp electrode
IDR	intradermal reaction	IgA	immunoglobulin A
IDS	infectious disease service	IgD	immunoglobulin D
IDU	idoxuridine	IGDE	idiopathic gait disorders of the elderly
	infectious disease unit	IGDM	infant of gestational diabetic mother
IDV	intermittent demand ventilation	IgE	immunoglobulin E
IDVC	indwelling venous catheter	IGF-I	insulin-like growth factor
IE	immunoelectrophoresis	IgG	immunoglobulin G
	induced emesis	IGIM	immune globulin intramuscular
	infective endocarditis		
	inner ear	IGIV	immune globulin intravenous
	international unit (European abbreviation)		
I & E	ingress and egress (tubes)	IgM	immunoglobulin M
i.e.	that is	IGR	intrauterine growth retardation
I:E ratio	inspiratory to expiratory time ratio	IGT	impaired glucose tolerance
I&E	internal and external		
IEC	inpatient exercise center	IH	indirect hemagglutination
IEF	isoelectric focusing		infectious hepatitis
IEM	immune electron microscopy		inguinal hernia
		IHA	immune hemolytic anemia
	inborn errors of metabolism		indirect hemagglutination
			infusion hepatic arteriography
IEP	immunoelectrophoresis		
	Individualized Education Plan	IHC	immobilization hypercalcemia
IET	infantile estropia		inner hair cell (in cochlea)
IF	idiopathic flushing		
	ifosfamide	IHD	intraheptic duct (ule)
	immunofluorescence		ischemic heart disease
	interferon	IHH	idiopathic hypogonadotrophic hypogonadism
	intermaxillary fixation		
	internal fixation		

IHO	idiopathic hypertrophic osteoarthropathy
IHR	inguinal hernia repair
IHS	Indian Health Service
	Iodiopathic Headache Score
IHs	iris hamartomas
IHSA	iodinated human serum albumin
IHSS	idiopathic hypertrophic subaortic stenosis
IHT	insulin hypoglycemia test
IHW	inner heel wedge
IIA	internal iliac artery
IICP	increased intracranial pressure
IICU	infant intensive care unit
IJ	ileojejunal
	internal jugular
I&J	insight and judgment
IJC	internal jugular catheter
IJD	inflammatory joint disease
IJR	idiojunctional rhythm
IJT	idiojunctional tachycardia
IJV	internal jugular vein
IK	immobilized knee
	interstitial keratitis
IL	immature lungs
	interleukin (1, 2, and 3)
	intralesional
	Intralipid®
ILA	indicated low forceps
ILBBB	incomplete left bundle branch block
ILBW	infant, low birth weight
ILD	intermediate density lipoproteins
	interstitial lung disease
	ischemic leg disease
ILE	infantile lobar emphysema
ILF	indicated low forceps
ILFC	immature living female child
ILM	internal limiting membrane
ILMC	immature living male child
ILMI	inferolateral myocardial infarct

ILVEN	inflammatory linear verrucal epidermal nevus
IM	infectious mononucleosis
	intermetatarsal
	internal medicine
	intramedullary
	intramuscular
IMA	inferior mesenteric artery
	internal mammary artery
IMAC	ifosfamide, mesna uroprotection, doxorubicin, and cisplatin
IMAG	internal mammary artery graft
IMB	intermenstrual bleeding
IMC	intermittent catheterization
	intramedullary catheter
IMCU	intermediate care unit
IME	independent medical examination
IMF	ifosfamide, mesna uroprotection, methotrexate, and fluorouracil
	immobilization mandibular fracture
	intermaxillary fixation
IMG	internal medicine group (group practices)
IMGU	insulin-mediated glucose uptake
IMH test	indirect microhemagglutination test
IMI	imipramine
	inferior myocardial infarction
IMIG	intramuscular immunoglobulin
IMLC	incomplete mitral leaflet closure
IMN	internal mammary (lymph) node
IMP	impacted
	important
	impression
	improved

IMRA	immunoradiometric assay	INO	internuclear ophthal-
IMS	incurred in military		moplegia
	service	INDO	indomethacin
IMT	inspiratory muscle	inpt	inpatient
	training	INR	international normalized
IMU	intermediate medicine		ratio (for anticoagulant
	unit		monitoring)
IMV	inferior mesenteric vein	INS	insurance
	intermittent mandatory	INST	instrumental delivery
	ventilation	INT	intermittent needle
	intermittent mechanical		therapy
	ventilation		internal
IMVP-16	ifosfamide, mesna	Int mon	internal monitor
	uroprotection,	INTERP	interpretation
	methotrexate, and	intol	intolerance
	etoposide	int-rot	internal rotation
IN	intranasal	int trx	intermittent traction
In	inches	intub	intubation
	indium	inver	inversion
INC	incisal	I&O	intake and output
	incision	IO	inferior oblique
	incomplete		initial opening
	incontinent		intraocular pressure
	increase	IOA	intact on admission
	inside-the-needle catheter	IOC	intern on call
Inc Spir	incentive spirometer		intraoperative
IND	induced		cholangiogram
	Investigational New Drug	IOCG	intraoperative
	(application)		cholangiogram
INDM	infant of nondiabetic	IOD	interorbital distance
	mother	IODM	infant of diabetic mother
INEX	inexperienced	IOF	intraocular fluid
INF	infant	IOFB	intraocular foreign body
	infarction	IOFNA	intraoperative fine needle
	infected		aspiration
	inferior	IOH	idiopathic orthostatic
	information		hypotension
	infused	IOI	intraosseous infusion
	infusion	IOL	intraocular lens
	intravenous nutritional	IOLI	intraocular lens
	fluid		implantation
INFC	infected	ION	ischemic optic neuropathy
	infection	IONIS	indirect optic nerve injury
ING	inguinal		syndrome
✔ ing	checking	IONTO	iontophoresis
INH	isoniazid	IOP	intraocular pressure
inj	injection	IOR	ideas of reference
	injury	IORT	intraoperative radiation
INK	injury not known		therapy

IOS	intraoperative sonography	IPMI	inferoposterior myocardial infarct
IOT	intraocular tension		
IOV	initial office visit	IPN	infantile periarteritis nodosa
IP	incubation period		
	individualized plan		intern's progress note
	in plaster	IPOF	immediate postoperative fitting
	interphalangeal		
	intraperitoneal	IPOP	immediate postoperative prosthesis
I/P	iris/pupil		
IP3	inositol triphosphate	IPP	inflatable penile prosthesis
IPA	independent practice association		
		IPPA	inspection, palpation, percussion, and auscultation
	interpleural analgesia		
	invasive pulmonary aspergillosis		
		IPPB	intermittent positive pressure breathing
	isopropyl alcohol		
IPAP	inspiratory positive airway pressure	IPPF	immediate postoperative prosthetic fitting
IPB	infrapopliteal bypass	IPPI	interruption of pregnancy for psychiatric indication
IPC	indirect pulp cavity		
	intermittent pneumatic compression (boots)		
		IPPV	intermittent positive pressure ventilation
IPCD	infantile polycystic disease		
IPCK	infantile polycystic kidney (disease)	IPS	infundibular pulmonic stenosis
IPD	immediate pigment darkening	IPSF	immediate postsurgical fitting
	inflammatory pelvic disease	IPSID	immunoproliferative small intestinal disease
	intermittent peritoneal dialysis	iPTH	parathyroid hormone by radioimmunoassay
	interpupillary distance	IPTX	intermittent pelvic traction
IPF	idiopathic pulmonary fibrosis	IPV	inactivated poliovirus vaccine
IPFD	intrapartum fetal distress	IPVC	interpolated premature ventricular contraction
IPG	impedance plethysmography		
		IPW	interphalangeal width
	individually polymerized grass	IQ	intelligence quotient
		IR	inferior rectus
IPH	idiopathic pulmonary hemosiderosis		infrared
			internal reduction
	interphalangeal		internal rotation
	intraparenchymal hemorrhage	I&R	insertion and removal
		IRA-EEA	ileorectal anastomoses with end-to-end anastomosis
IPJ	interphalangeal joint		
IPK	intractable plantar keratosis		
		IRB	Institutional Review Board
IPM	intrauterine pressure monitor	IRBBB	incomplete right bundle branch block

IRBC	immature red blood cell	ISDN	isosorbide dinitrate
	irradiated red blood cells	ISG	immune serum globulin
IRBP	interphotoreceptor		(immune globulin)
	retinoid-binding protein	ISH	isolated systolic
IRC	indirect radionuclide		hypertension
	cystography	ISHT	isolated systolic
IRCU	intensive respiratory care		hypertension
	unit	ISI	International Sensitivity
IRDS	idiopathic respiratory		Index
	distress syndrome	ISMA	infantile spinal muscular
	infant respiratory distress		atrophy
	syndrome	ISMO®	isosorbide mononitrate
	insulin-resistant diabetes	ISO	isolette
	mellitus		isoproterenol
IRH	intraretinal hemorrhage	ISOE	isoetharine
IRMA	immunoradiometric assay	ISQ	as before; continue on (*in*
	intraretinal microvascular		*status quo*)
	abnormalities	ISS	idiopathic short stature
IROS	ipsilateral routing of		Injury Severity Score
	signals		Individual Self-Rating
IRR	intrarenal reflux		Scale
IRRC	Institutional Research		irritable stomach
	Review Committee		syndrome
irreg	irregular		Integrated Summary of
IRR			Safety
HYDRO	irreversible hydrocolloid	IS10S	10% invert sugar in 0.9%
IRS	Information and Referral		sodium chloride
	Society		injection (saline)
IRT	immunoreactive trypsin	IST	insulin sensitivity test
IRV	inspiratory reserve		insulin shock therapy
	volume	ISU	intermediate surgical unit
	inverse ratio ventilation	ISW	interstitial water
IS	incentive spirometer	IS10W	10% invert sugar injection
	induced sputum		(in water)
	intercostal space	ISWI	incisional surgical wound
	inventory of systems		infection
	ipecac syrup	IT	individual therapy
I/S	instruct/supervise		inferior-temporal
ISA	intrinsic sympathomimetic		Inhalation Therapist
	activity		inhalation therapy
ISB	incentive spirometry		intensive therapy
	breathing		intermittent traction
ISC	infant servo-control		intertuberous
	infant skin control		intrathecal (dangerous)
	isolette servo-control		intratracheal (dangerous,
ISCs	irreversible sickle cells		could be interupted as
ISD	inhibited sexual desire		intrathecal)
	initial sleep disturbance	ITA	individual treatment
	isosorbide dinitrate		assessment

ITAG	internal thoracic artery graft		term birth, cesarean section
ITB	iliotibial band	IUP,TBLC	intrauterine pregnancy, term birth, living child
ITC	Incontinence Treatment Center	IUR	intrauterine retardation
ITCP	idiopathic thrombocytopenic purpura	IUT	intrauterine transfusion
		IUTD	immunizations up to date
ITCU	intensive thoracic cardiovascular unit	IV	four
			interview
ITE	insufficient therapeutic effect		intravenous (i.v.)
			symbol for class 4 controlled substances
	in-the-ear (hearing aid)	IVA	Intervir-A
ITGV	intrathoracic gas volume	IVAP	implantable vascular access device
ITP	idiopathic thrombocytopenic purpura	IVBAT	intravascular bronchoalveolar tumor
	interim treatment plan	IVC	inferior vena cava
ITPA	Illinois Test of Psycholinguistic Ability		inspiratory vital capacity
			intravenous cholangiogram
ITRA	itraconazole		
ITSCU	infant-toddler special care unit		intraventricular catheter
		IVCD	intraventricular conduction defect
ITT	identical twins (raised) together	IVD	intervertebral disk
			intravenous drip
	insulin tolerance test	IVDA	intravenous drug abuse
ITU	infant-toddler unit	IVDSA	intravenous digital subtraction angiography
ITVAD	indwelling transcutaneous vascular access device		
		IVDU	intravenous drug user
IU	international unit (this is a dangerous abbreviation as it is read as intravenous)	IVF	in vitro fertilization
			intravenous fluid(s)
		IVFA	intravenous fluorescein angiography
IUC	intrauterine catheter	IVFE	intravenous fat emulsion
IUCD	intrauterine contraceptive device	IVF-ET	in vitro fertilization-embryo transfer
IUD	intrauterine death	IVFT	intravenous fetal transfusion
	intrauterine device		
IUDR	idoxuridine	IVGTT	intravenous glucose tolerance test
IUFB	intrauterine foreign body	IVH	intravenous hyperalimentation
IUFD	intrauterine fetal death		
	intrauterine fetal distress		intraventricular hemorrhage
IUGR	intrauterine growth retardation	IVIG	intravenous immunoglobulin
IUI	intrauterine insemination		
IUP	intrauterine pregnancy	IVJC	intervertebral joint complex
IUPC	intrauterine pressure catheter		
IUPD	intrauterine pregnancy delivered		
IUP,TBCS	intrauterine pregnancy,		

IVL	intravenous lock	JAMG	juvenile autoimmune myasthenia gravis
IVLBW	infant of very low birth weight	JAR	junior assistant resident
IVOX	intravascular oxygenator	JARAN	junior assistant resident admission note
IVP	intravenous push	JBE	Japanese B encephalitis
	intravenous pyelogram	JC	junior clinicians (medical students)
IVPB	intravenous piggyback		
IVPU	intravenous push	JCAHO	Joint Commission on Accreditation of Healthcare Organizations
IVR	idioventricular rhythm		
	intravenous retrograde		
	intravenous rider		
IVRAP	intravenous retrograde access port	JD	jaundice
		JDG	jugulodigastric
IVRG	intravenous retrograde	JDMS	juvenile dermatomyositis
IVRO	intraoral vertical ramus osteotomy	JE	Japanese encephalitis
		JEB	junctional escape beat
IVS	intraventricular septum	JER	junctional escape rhythm
	irritable voiding syndrome	JET	junctional ectopic tachycardia
IVSD	intraventricular septal defect		
		JF	joint fluid
IVSE	interventricular septal excursion	JFS	Jewish Family Service
		JHR	Jarisch-Herxheimer reaction
IVSS	intravenous Soluset®		
IVT	intravenous transfusion	JI	jejunoileal
IVTTT	intravenous tolbutamide tolerance test	JIB	jejunoileal bypass
		JIS	juvenile idiopathic scoliosis
IVU	intravenous urography		
IWI	inferior wall infarction	JJ	jaw jerk
IWL	insensible water loss	JLP	juvenile laryngeal papillomatosis
IWMI	inferior wall myocardial infarct		
		JM-9	iproplatin
IWML	idiopathic white matter lesion	JMS	junior medical student
		JND	just noticeable difference
IWT	impacted wisdom teeth	jnt	joint
		JODM	juvenile onset diabetes mellitus
		JOMAC	judgment, orientation, memory, affect, and calculation
		JOMACI	judgment, orientation, memory, abstraction, and calculation intact
	J		
		JP	Jackson-Pratt (drain)
			Jobst pump
			joint protection
J	jejunostomy	JPB	junctional premature beats
	Jewish	JP➤BS	Jackson-Pratt to bulb suction
	joint		
	joule		
	juice		
Jack	jacknife position		

JPC	junctional premature contraction		Ka	first order absorption constant in hr.$^{-1}$
JPS	joint position sense		KAB	knowledge, attitude, and behavior
JPTS	juvenile tropical pancreatitis syndrome		K-ABC	Kaufman Assessment Battery for Children
JR	junctional rhythm			
JRA	juvenile rheumatoid arthritis		KABINS	knowledge, attitude, behavior, and improvement in nutritional status
JRAN	junior resident admission note			
Jr BF	junior baby food		KAFO	knee-ankle-foot orthosis
JRC	joint replacement center		KAO	knee-ankle orthosis
JT	jejunostomy tube		KAS	Katz Adjustment Scale
	joint		KASH	knowledge, abilities, skills, and habits
	junctional tachycardia			
JTF	jejunostomy tube feeding		kat	katal
JTP	joint projection		K-A units	King-Armstrong units
J-Tube	jejunostomy tube		KB	ketone bodies
juv.	juvenile		KC	keratoconjunctivitis
JV	jugular vein			knees to chest
JVC	jugular venous catheter			Korean conflict
JVD	jugular venous distention		kcal	kilocalorie
JVP	jugular venous pressure		kCi	kilocurie
	jugular venous pulsation		KCl	potassium chloride
	jugular venous pulse		KCS	keratoconjunctivitis sicca
JVPT	jugular venous pulse tracing		KD	Kawasaki's disease
				Keto Diastix®
JW	Jehovah's Witness			kidney donors
Jx	joint			knee disarticulation
JXG	juvenile xanthogranuloma		Kd	kilodalton
			KDA	known drug allergies
			KDU	Kidney Dialysis Unit
			KE	first order elimination rate constant in hr.$^{-1}$

K

			KED	Kendrick extrication device
			k_{el}	elimination rate constant
			KET	ketoconazole
K	kelvin		17 Keto	17 ketosteroids
	potassium		KF	kidney function
	thousand		KFAO	knee-foot-ankle orthosis
	vitamin K		KFD	Kyasanur Forrest disease
K_1	phytonadione		KFR	Kayser-Fleischer ring
K_3	menadione		kg	kilogram
K_4	menadiol sodium diphosphate		KGC	Keflin®, gentamicin, and carbenicillin
17K	17-ketosteroids		K24H	potassium, urine 24 hour
KA	keratoacanthoma		KI	karyopyknotic index
	ketoacidosis			knee immobilizer

	potassium iodide	KV	kilovolt
KID	keratitis, ichthyosis, and deafness (syndrome)	KVO	keep vein open
		KVP	kilovolt peak
kilo	kilogram	KW	Keith-Wagener
KISS	saturated solution of potassium iodide		(ophthalmoscopic finding, graded I-IV)
KIT	Kahn Intelligence Test		Kimmelstiel-Wilson
KJ	kilojoule	KWB	Keith, Wagener, Barker
	knee jerk	K-wire	Kirschner wire
KK	knee kick		
KL-BET	Kleihauer-Betke		
KPE	Kemper phako-emulsification		
Kleb	*Klebsiella*		**L**
KLH	keyhole limpet hemocyanin		
K-Lor®	potassium chloride tablets		
KLS	kidneys, liver, and spleen	L	fifty
KM	kanamycin		left
$KMnO_4$	potassium permanganate		lente insulin
KN	knee		lingual
KNO	keep needle open		liter
KO	keep open		liver
	knee orthosis		lumbar
KOH	potassium hydroxide		lung
KOR	keep open rate	Ⓛ	left
KP	hot pack	$L_1...L_5$	lumbar nerve 1 through 5
	keratoprecipitate		lumbar vertebra 1 through 5
KPE	Kelman phacoemulsification		
Kr	krypton	LA	language age
KS	Kaposi's sarcoma		Latin American
17-KS	17-ketosteroids		left arm
KSA	knowledge, skills, and abilities		left atrial
			left atrium
KS/OI	Kaposi's sarcoma and opportunistic infections		local anesthesia
			long acting
KSR	potassium chloride sustained release (tablets)	L + A	light and accommodation
			living and active
KT	kidney transplant	LAA	left atrium and its appendage
	kinesiotherapy		
KTC	knee to chest	LAB	laboratory
KTP	potassium-titanyl--phosphate (laser)		left abdomen
		LAC	laceration
KTU	kidney transplant unit		long arm cast
KUB	kidney, ureter, and bladder	LACT-ART	lactate arterial
KUS	kidney(s), ureter(s), and spleen	LAD	left anterior descending
			left axis deviation

LADA	left anterior descending (coronary) artery		leucine acetylsalicylate
			long arm splint
LADCA	left anterior descending coronary artery		lymphadenopathy syndrome
LADD	left anterior descending diagonal		lymphangioscintigraphy
LAD-MIN	left axis deviation minimal	LASA	Linear Analogue Self-Assessment (scales)
LAE	left atrial enlargement		lipid-associated sialic acid
	long above elbow	L-ASP	asparaginase
LAF	laminar air flow	LAT	lateral
	Latin-American female		left anterior thigh
	low animal fat	LATCH	literature attached to chart
	lymphocyte-activating factor	lat.men.	lateral meniscectomy
		LATS	long-acting thyroid stimulator
LAFB	left anterior fascicular block	LAV	lymphadenopathy associated virus
LAG	lymphangiogram		
LAH	left anterior hemiblock	LAVA	laser-assisted vasal anastomosis
	left atrial hypertrophy		
LAHB	left anterior hemiblock	LAVH	laparoscopically assisted vaginal hysterectomy
LAK	lymphokine-activated killer		
		LAW	left atrial wall
LAL	left axillary line	LAX	laxative
	limulus amebocyte lysate	LB	large bowel
LAM	laminectomy		left breast
	laminogram		left buttock
	Latin-American male		live births
lam✔	laminectomy check		low back
LAMB	mucocutaneous lentigines, atrial myxoma, and blue nevus (syndrome)		lung biopsy
			lymphoid body
			pound
LANC	long arm navicular cast	L&B	left and below
LAN	lymphadenopathy	LBB	left breast biopsy
LAO	left anterior oblique	LBBB	left bundle branch block
LAP	laparoscopy	LBCD	left border of cardiac dullness
	laparotomy		
	left arterial pressure	LBD	large bile duct
	leucine amino peptidase		left border dullness
	leukocyte alkaline phosphatase	LBE	long below elbow
		LBH	length, breadth, and height
LAP-APPY	laparoscopic appendectomy		
		LBM	lean body mass
LAPMS	long arm posterior molded splint		loose bowel movement
		LBO	large bowel obstruction
LAPW	left atrial posterior wall	LBP	low back pain
LAQ	long arc quad		low blood pressure
LAR	left arm, reclining	LBQC	large base quad cane
LAS	laxative abuse syndrome	LBT	low back tenderness

	low back trouble
LBV	left brachial vein
LBW	lean body weight
	low birth weight
LC	left circumflex
	leisure counseling
	living children
	low calorie
	lung cancer
3LC	triple lumen catheter
LCA	Leber's congenital amaurosis
	left circumflex artery
	left coronary artery
	light contact assist
LCAT	lecithin cholesterol acyltransferase
LCB	left costal border
LCCA	left common carotid artery
	leukocytoclastic angiitis
LCCS	low cervical cesarean section
LCD	coal tar solution (*liquor carbonis detergens*)
	localized collagen dystrophy
	low calcium diet
LCE	left carotid endarterectomy
LCF	left circumflex
LCFA	long-chain fatty acid
LCFM	left circumflex marginal
LCGU	local cerebral glucose utilization
LCH	local city hospital
LCIS	lobular cancer *in situ*
LCL	lateral collateral ligament
LCLC	large cell lung carcinoma
LCM	left costal margin
	lymphocytic choriomeningitis
LCR	late cortical response
	late cutaneous reaction
	vincristine
LCS	low constant suction
	low continuous suction
LCSW	Licensed Clinical Social Worker

	low continuous wall suction
LCT	long chain triglyceride
	low cervical transverse
	lymphocytotoxicity
LCTD	low-calcium test diet
LCV	leucovorin
	low cervical vertical
LCX	left circumflex coronary artery
LD	labor and delivery
	lactic dehydrogenase (formerly LDH)
	last dose
	learning disability
	learning disorder
	left deltoid
	Legionnaire's disease
	lethal dose
	levodopa
	Licensed Dietician
	liver disease
	living donor
	loading dose
	long dwell
LDB	Legionnaires disease bacterium
LDCOC	low-dose combination oral contraceptive
LDDS	local dentist
LDEA	left deviation of electrical axis
LDH	lactic dehydrogenase
LDIH	left direct inguinal hernia
LDL	low-density lipoprotein
LDLC	low-density lipoprotein cholesterol
L-dopa	levodopa
LDR	labor, delivery, and recovery
	length-to-diameter ratio
LDR/P	labor, delivery, recovery, and postpartum
LDT	left dorsotransverse
LDUB	long double upright brace
LDV	laser Doppler velocimetry
LE	left ear
	left eye
	lens extraction

	live embryo	LFT	latex flocculation test
	lower extremities		left fronto-transverse
	lupus erythematosus		liver function tests
LEA	lumbar epidural anesthesia	LFU	limit flocculation unit
		LG	large
LED	lupus erythematosus disseminatus		laryngectomy
			left gluteal
LEHPZ	lower esophageal high pressure zone	LGA	large for gestational age
			left gastric artery
LEJ	ligation of the esophagogastric junction	LGI	lower gastrointestinal (series)
		LGL	Lown-Ganong-Levine (syndrome)
LEM	lateral eye movements		
	light electron microscope	LGM	left gluteus medius
LEP	lower esophageal pressure	LGN	lobular glomerulonephritis
LEP 2	leptospirosis 2	LGS	Lennox-Gastaut syndrome
LE prep	lupus erythematosus preparation	LGV	lymphagranuloma venerum
L-ERX	leukoerythroblastic reaction	LH	left hand
			left hyperphoria
LES	local excitatory state		luteinizing hormone
	lower esophageal sphincter	LHA	left hepatic artery
		LHF	left heart failure
	lupus erythematosus systemic	LHG	left hand grip
		LHH	left homonymous hemianopsia
LESP	lower esophageal sphincter pressure		
		LHL	left hemisphere lesions
LET	linear energy transfer	LHP	left hemiparesis
LEV	levator muscle	LHR	leukocyte histamine release
LF	Lassa fever		
	left foot	LHRH	luteinizing hormone-releasing hormone (hypothalamic)
	low fat		
	low forceps		
	low frequency	LHRT	leukocyte histamine release test
LFA	left femoral artery		
	left forearm	LHS	left hand side
	left fronto-anterior	LHT	left hypertropia
	low friction arthroplasty	LI	lactose intolerance
LFC	living female child		large intestine
	low fat and cholesterol		learning impaired
LFD	lactose-free diet	Li	lithium
	low fat diet	LIA	left iliac artery
	low fiber diet	LIB	left in bottle
	low forceps delivery	LIC	left iliac crest
LFGNR	lactose fermenting gram-negative rod		left internal carotid
			leisure interest class
LFL	left frontolateral	LICA	left internal carotid artery
LFP	left frontoposterior	LICD	lower intestinal Crohn's disease
LFS	liver function series		

LICM	left intercostal margin
Li_2CO_3	lithium carbonate
LICS	left intercostal space
Lido	lidocaine
LIF	left iliac fossa
	liver (migration) inhibitory factor
	left index finger
LIG	ligament
LIH	left inguinal hernia
LIHA	low impulsiveness, high anxiety
LIJ	left internal jugular
LILA	low impulsiveness, low anxiety
LIMA	left internal mammary artery (graft)
LING	lingual
LIO	left inferior oblique
LIP	lithium-induced polydipsia
	lymphocytic interstitial pneumonia
LIPV	left inferior pulmonary vein
LIQ	liquid
	lower inner quadrant
LIR	left iliac region
	left inferior rectus
LIS	left intercostal space
	low intermittent suction
LISS	low ionic strength saline
LITH	lithotomy
LIV	left innominate vein
LIVC	left inferior vena cava
LIVPRO	liver profile
LIWS	low intermittent wall suction
LJM	limited joint mobility
LK	lamellar keratoplasty
	left kidney
LKA	Lazare-Klerman-Armour (Personality Inventory)
LKKS	liver, kidneys, spleen
LKS	liver, kidneys, spleen
LKSB	liver, kidneys, spleen, and bladder
LKSNP	liver, kidney, and spleen not palpable

L⟍ M K O S⟋ T	liver, kidneys, and spleen negative, no masses, or tenderness
LL	large lymphocyte
	left lateral
	left leg
	left lower
	left lung
	lower lid
	lower lip
	lower lobe
	lumbar laminectomy
	lumbar length
	lymphocytic leukemia
	lymphoblastic lymphoma
L&L	lids and lashes
LL2	limb lead two
LLA	limulus lysate assay
LLB	left lateral border
	long leg brace
LLC	laparoscopic laser cholecystectomy
	long leg cast
LLBCD	left lower border of cardiac dullness
LLD	left lateral decubitus
	left length discrepancy
LLE	left lower extremity
LLFG	long leg fiberglas (cast)
LL-GXT	low-level graded exercise test
LLL	left lower lid
	left lower lobe (lung)
LLLE	lower lid left eye
LLLNR	left lower lobe, no rales
LLO	Legionella-like organism
LLOD	lower lid, right eye
LLOS	lower lid, left eye
LLP	long leg plaster
LLQ	left lower quadrant (abdomen)
LLR	left lateral rectus
LLRE	lower lid, right eye
LLS	lazy leukocyte syndrome
LLSB	left lower sternal border
LLT	left lateral thigh
LLWC	long leg walking cast
LLX	left lower extremity

LM	left main		lumbar orthosis
L/M	liters per minute	LOA	leave of absence
LMA	left mentoanterior		left occiput anterior
	liver membrane		looseness of associations
	autoantibody		lysis of adhesions
LMB	Laurence-Moon-Biedl	LOB	loss of balance
	syndrome	LOC	laxative of choice
LMC	living male child		level of care
LMCA	left main coronary artery		level of comfort
	left middle cerebral artery		level of consciousness
LMCAT	left middle cerebral artery		local
	thrombosis		loss of consciousness
LMCL	left midclavicular line	LOCM	low-osmolality contrast
LMD	local medical doctor		media
	low molecular weight	LOD	line of duty
	dextran	LOIH	left oblique inguinal
LME	left mediolateral		hernia
	episiotomy	LOI	Leyton Obsessional
LMEE	left middle ear		Inventory
	exploration	LOL	left occipitolateral
LMF	left middle finger		little old lady
L/min	liters per minute	LOM	left otitis media
LML	left medial lateral		limitation of motion
	left middle lobe		loss of motion
LMLE	left mediolateral		low-osmolar (contrast)
	episiotomy		media
LMM	lentigo maligna melanoma	LOMSA	left otitis media,
LMP	last menstrual period		suppurative, acute
	left mentoposterior	LOMSC	left otitis media,
LMR	left medial rectus		suppurative, chronic
LMS	lateral medullary	LoNa	low sodium
	syndrome	LOP	leave on pass
LMT	left main trunk		left occiput posterior
	left mentotransverse	LOQ	lower outer quadrant
LMWD	low molecular weight	LORS-I	Level of Rehabilitation
	dextran		Scale-I
LMWH	low molecular weight	LOS	length of stay
	heparin	LOT	left occiput transverse
LN	left nostril (nare)		Licensed Occupational
	lymph nodes		Therapist
LN_2	liquid nitrogen	LOV	loss of vision
LNCs	lymph node cells	LOZ	lozenge
LND	light-near dissociation	LP	light perception
	lymph node dissection		low protein
LNG	levonorgestrel		lumbar puncture
LNMP	last normal menstrual	L/P	lactate-pyruvate ratio
	period	LPA	left pulmonary artery
LO	lateral oblique (x-ray	L-PAM	melphalan
	view)	LPC	laser photocoagulation

	Licensed Professional Counselor	L&R gtt	Levophed® and Regitine® drip (infusion)
LPCC	Licensed Professional Certified Counselor	LRI	lower respiratory infection
LPc̄P	light perception with projection	LRM	left radical mastectomy
LPD	leiomyomatosis peritonealis disseminata	LRMP	last regular menstrual period
		LRND	left radical neck dissection
	low protein diet	LRO	long range objective
	luteal phase defect	LRQ	lower right quadrant
	luteal phase deficiency	LRS	lactated Ringer's solution
LPEP	left pre-ejection period	LRT	lower respiratory tract
lpf	low-power field	LRTI	lower respiratory tract infection
LPF	liver plasma flow	LRV	left renal vein
LPFB	left posterior fascicular block		log reduction value
LPH	left posterior hemiblock	LRZ	lorazepam
LPI	laser peripheral iridectomy	LS	left side
			legally separated
LPL	lipoprotein lipase		Leigh's syndrome
LPLND	laparoscopic pelvic lymph node dissection		liver scan
			liver-spleen
LPM	liters per minute		low salt
LPN	Licensed Practical Nurse		lumbosacral
LPO	left posterior oblique	L/S	lecithin-sphingomyelin ratio
	light perception only	L&S	ligation and stripping
LPPC	leukocyte-poor packed cells	L5-S1	lumbar fifth vertebra to sacral first vertebra
LPS	last Pap smear	LSA	left sacrum anterior
	lipopolysaccharide		lipid-bound sialic acid
LPT	Licensed Physical Therapist		lymphosarcoma
		LSB	left sternal border
LPTN	Licensed Psychiatric Technical Nurse		local standby
			lumbar spinal block
LR	labor room		lumbar sympathetic block
	lactated Ringer's (injection)	LS BPS	laparoscopic bilateral partial salpingectomy
	lateral rectus	LSC	late systolic click
	left-right		lichen simplex chronicus
	light reflex	LSCA	left scapuloanterior
L→R	left to right	LSCP	left scapuloposterior
LR1A	labor room 1A	LSD	low salt diet
LRA	left radial artery		lysergide
LRD	living related donor	LSE	local side effects
	living renal donor	LSF	low saturated fat
LREH	low renin essential hypertension	LSFA	low saturated fatty acid (diet)
LRF	left rectus femoris	LSKM	liver-spleen-kidney-megalgia

LSL	left sacrolateral	LTFU	long-term follow-up
	left short leg (brace)	LTG	long-term goal
LSM	late systolic murmur	LTGA	left transposition of great
LSO	left salpingo-		artery
	oophorectomy	LTL	laparoscopic tubal ligation
	left superior oblique	LTM	long-term memory
	lumbosacral orthosis	LTOT	long-term oxygen therapy
LSP	left sacrum posterior	LTP	laser trabeculoplasty
	liver-specific (membrane)		long-term plan
	lipoprotein	LTR	long terminal repeats
L–Spar	Elspar (asparaginase)	LTS	laparoscopic tubal
L-SPINE	lumbar spine		sterilization
LSR	left superior rectus	LTT	lactose tolerance test
L/S ratio	lecithin/sphingomyelin		lymphocyte transforma-
	ratio		tion test
LSS	liver-spleen scan	LTUI	low transverse uterine
LST	left sacrum transverse		incision
LSTC	laparoscopic tubal	LTV	long term variability
	coagulation		Luche tumor virus
LSTL	laparoscopic tubal ligation	LTVC	long-term venous catheter
L's & T's	lines and tubes	LU	left ureteral
LSU	life support unit		living unit
LSV	left subclavian vein		Lutheran
LSVC	left superior vena cava	L & U	lower and upper
LT	laboratory technician	LUA	left upper arm
	left	LUD	left uterine displacement
	left thigh	LUE	left upper extremity
	leukotrienes	Lues I	primary syphilis
	Levin tube	LUL	left upper lid
	light		left upper lobe (lung)
	light touch	LUOB	left upper outer buttock
	low transverse	LUOQ	left upper outer quadrant
	lumbar traction	LUQ	left upper quadrant
	lymphotoxin	LURD	living unrelated donor
LTA	laryngeal tracheal	LUS	lower uterine segment
	anesthesia	LUSB	left upper sternal border
	local tracheal anesthesia	LUX	left upper extremity
LTB	laparoscopic tubal	LV	leave
	banding		left ventricle
	laryngotracheo-bronchitis		leucovorin
LTB$_4$	leukotriene B$_4$	LVA	left ventricular aneurysm
LTC	left to count	LVC	low viscosity cement
	long-term care	LVAD	left ventricular assist
LTC$_4$	leukotriene C$_4$		device
LTC-101	long-term care form-101	L-VAM	leuprolide acetate,
LTCF	long-term care facility		vinblastine,
LTCS	low transverse cesarean		doxorubicin, and
	section		mitomycin
LTD	largest tumor dimension		

LVAT	left ventricular activation time		myocardial ischemia
		LVSP	left ventricular systolic pressure
LVD	left ventricular dysfunction		
		LVSWI	left ventricular stroke work index
LVDP	left ventricular diastolic pressure		
		LVV	left ventricular volume
LVDV	left ventricular diastolic volume		live varicella vaccine
		LVW	left ventricular wall
LVE	left ventricular enlargement	LVWI	left ventricular work index
LVEDP	left ventricular end diastolic pressure	LVWMA	left ventricular wall motion abnormality
LVEDV	left ventricular end diastolic volume	LVWMI	left ventricular wall motion index
LVEF	left ventricular ejection fraction	LW	living will
		L & W	Lee and White (coagulation)
LVEP	left ventricular end pressure		living and well
LVESVI	left ventricular end systolic volume index	LWCT	Lee-White clotting time
		LWBS	left without being seen
LVET	left ventricular ejection time	LWC	leave without consent
		LWOT	left without treatment
LVF	left ventricular failure	LWP	large whirlpool
LVFP	left ventricular filling pressure	lx	larynx
			lower extremity
LVG	left ventrogluteal	LXC	laxative of choice
LVH	left ventricular hypertrophy	LXT	left exotropia
		LYG	lymphomatoid granulomatosis
LVIDd	left ventricle internal dimension diastole		
		LYM	lymphocytes
LVIDs	left ventricle internal dimension systole	lymphs	lymphocytes
		LYS	large yellow soft (stools)
LVL	left vastus lateralis		lysine
LVMM	left ventricular muscle mass	lytes	electrolytes (Na, K, Cl, etc.)
LVN	Licensed Visiting Nurse Licensed Vocational Nurse	LZP	lorazepam
LVOP	left ventricular outflow tract		
LVOT	left ventricular outflow tract		
LVP	large volume parenteral left ventricular pressure		**M**
LVPW	left ventricular posterior wall		
		M	male
LVR	leucovorin		marital
LVSEMI	left ventricular subendocardial		married
			mass

101

		MAC	macrocytic erythrocytes
	medial		macula
	memory		maximal allowable
	meta		concentration
	meter (m)		membrane attack complex
	mild		methotrexate,
	million		dactinomycin, and
	minimum		cyclophosphamide
	molar		mid-arm circumference
	Monday		minimum alveolar
	monocytes		concentration
	mother		monitored anesthesia care
	mouth		*Mycobacterium avium*
	murmur		complex
	muscle	MACC	methotrexate,
	myopia		doxorubicin,
	myopic		cyclophosphamide, and
	thousand		lomustine
Ⓜ	murmur	MACCC	Master Arts, Certified
M₁	first mitral sound		Clinical Competence
M1	left mastoid	MACOP-B	methotrexate,
M1 to M7	categories of acute		doxorubicin,
	nonlymphoblastic		cyclophosphamide,
	leukemia		vincristine, prednisone,
M²	square meters (body		and bleomycin
	surface)	MACRO	macrocytes
M2	right mastoid	MACTAR	McMaster-Toronto
M-2	vincristine, carmustine,		Arthritis Patient
	cyclophosphamide,		Reference (Disability
	melphalan, and		Questionnaire)
	prednisone	MAD	mind altering drugs
MA	machine	MADRS	Montgomery-Asburg
	Master of Arts		Depression Rating
	medical assistance		Scale
	medical authorization	MAE	moves all extremities
	menstrual age	MAES	moves all extremities
	mental age		slowly
	Mexican American	MAEEW	moves all extremities
	microaneurysms		equally well
	Miller-Abbott (tube)	MAEW	moves all extremities well
	milliamps	MAFAs	movement-associated fetal
	monoclonal antibodies		(heart rate)
	motorcycle accident		accelerations
M/A	mood and/or affect	MAFO	molded ankle/foot
MA-1	Bennett volume ventilator		orthosis
MAA	macroaggregates of	mag cit	magnesium citrate
	albumin	mag sulf	magnesium sulfate
Mab	monoclonal antibody	MAHA	macroangiopathic
MABP	mean arterial blood		hemolytic anemia
	pressure		

MAI	maximal aggregation index			maternal
				maternity
	minor acute illness			mature
	Mycobacterium avium-intracellulare			medication administration team
MAID	mesna, doxorubicin (Adriamycin®), ifosfamide, and dacarbazine			multifocal atrial tachycardia
			MAU	microalbuminuria
			MAVR	mitral and aortic valve replacement
MAL	malignant			
	midaxillary line		max	maxillary
malig	malignant			maximal
MALT	mucosa-associated lymphoid tissue		MB	buccal margin
				Mallory body
MAM	monitored administration of medication			muscle band
			M-BACOD	methotrexate, calcium leucovorin, bleomycin, doxorubicin, cyclophosphamide, vincristine, and dexamethasone
MAMC	mid-arm muscle circumference			
Mammo	mammography			
m-AMSA	amsacrine			
MAN	malignancy associated neutropenia		MBC	maximum bladder capacity
Mand	mandibular			maximum breathing capacity
MANOVA	multivariate analysis of variance			methotrexate, bleomycin, and cisplatin
MAO	maximum acid output			minimal bactericidal concentration
MAOI	monoamine oxidase inhibitor			
MAP	mean airway pressure		MB-CK	a creatinine kinase isoenzyme
	mean arterial pressure		MBEST	modulus blipped echo-planar single-pulse technique
	mitomycin, doxorubicin, and cisplatin			
MAPS	make a picture story		MBD	minimal brain damage
	megaloblastic anemia of pregnancy			minimal brain dysfunction
			MBE	medium below elbow
MAR	medication administration record		MBF	meat base formula
				myocardial blood flow
MARE	manual active-resistive exercise		MBFC	medial brachial fascial compartment
MARSA	methicillin-aminoglycoside-resistant *Staphylococcus aureus*		MBI	methylene blue installation
			MBL	menstrual blood loss
MAS	meconium aspiration syndrome		MBM	mother's breast milk
			MBNW	multiple-breath nitrogen washout
	mobile arm support		MBO	mesiobuccal occulsion
MAST	mastectomy		MBP	major basic protein
	military antishock trousers			
MAT	manual arts therapy			

	malignant brachial plexopathy	MCLNS	mucocutaneous lymph node syndrome
MBq	megabecquerels	MCMI	Million Clinical Multiaxial Inventory
MBS	modified barium swallow		
MBT	maternal blood type	mcmol	micromoles
MC	male child	MCP	metacarpophalangeal joint metoclopramide
	metatarso - cuneiform		
	mitoxantrone and cytarabine	MCR	myocardial revascularization
	mixed cellularity	MCS	microculture and sensitivity
	molluscum contagiosum		
	monocomponent highly purified pork insulin	MCSA	minimal cross-sectional area
	mouth care	M-CSF	macrophage colony-stimulating factor
m + c	morphine and cocaine		
MCA	megestrol, cyclophospha- mide, and doxorubicin	MCT	manual cervical traction mean circulation time medium chain triglyceride medullary carcinoma of the thyroid
	middle cerebral aneurysm		
	middle cerebral artery		
	monoclonal antibodies		
	motorcycle accident	MCTC	metrizamide computed tomography cisternogram
	multichannel analyzer		
McB pt	McBurney's point		
MCC	midstream clean-catch	MCTD	mixed connective tissue disease
MCCU	mobile coronary care unit		
MCD	minimal change disease	MCU	micturating cystourethro- gram
MCDT	mast cell degranulation test		
		MCV	mean corpuscular volume
mcg	microgram (μg)	MD	maintenance dialysis maintenance dose major depression mammary dysplasia manic depression medical doctor mediodorsal mental deficiency movement disorder multiple dose muscular dystrophy
MCG	magnetocardiogram magnetocardiography		
MCGN	minimal-change glomerular nephritis		
MCH	mean corpuscular hemoglobin microfibrillar collagen hemostat muscle contraction headache		
MCHC	mean corpuscular hemoglobin concentration	MD-50®	diatrizoate sodium injection 50%
		MDA	malondialdehyde manual dilation of the anus methylenedioxyamphet- amine motor discriminative acuity
mCi	millicurie		
MCL	medial collateral ligament midclavicular line midcostal line modified chest lead most comfortable listening level		
		MDC	medial dorsal cutaneous (nerve)

MDD	major depressive disorder		middle ear
	manic depressive disorder		myalgic encephalomyelitis
MDE	major depressive episode	M/E	myeloid-erythroid (ratio)
MDF	myocardial depressant	M&E	Mecholyl® and Eserine®
	factor	MEA-I	multiple endocrine
MDGF	macrophage-derived		adenomatosis type I
	growth factor	MEB	methylene blue
MDI	manic depressive illness	MEC	meconium
	metered dose inhaler		middle ear canals
	methylenedioxyindenes	MeCCNU	semustine
	multiple daily injection	MECG	maternal electrocardio-
	multiple dosage insulin		gram
MDIA	Mental Development	MeCP	methyl-CCNU,
	Index, Adjusted		cyclophosphamide, and
MDII	multiple daily insulin		prednisone
	injection	MED	medial
MDM	mid-diastolic murmur		median erythrocyte
	minor determinant mix		diameter
	(of penicillin)		medical
MDMA	methylenedioxy-		medication
	methamphetamine		medicine
	(ecstasy)		medium
MDP	methylene diphosphonate		minimal erythema dose
MDPI	maximum daily		minimum effective dose
	permissible intake	MEDAC	multiple endocrine
MDR	minimum daily		deficiency-autoimmune-
	requirement		candidiasis
	multi-drug resistance	MEDCO	Medcosonolator
MDS	maternal deprivation	MEDEX	medication administration
	syndrome		record
	myelodysplastic	MED-	Medical Literature
	syndromes	LARS	Analysis and Retrieval
MDSU	medical day stay unit		System
MDT	multidisciplinary team	MEE	maintenance energy
MDTM	multidisciplinary team		expenditure
	meeting		measured energy
MDTP	multidisciplinary		expenditure
	treatment plan		middle ear effusion
MDUO	myocardial disease of	MEF	maximum expired flow
	unknown origin		rate
MDV	Marek's disease virus		middle ear fluid
	multiple dose vial	MEFR	mid expiratory flow rate
MDY	month, date, and year	MEFV	maximum expiratory
ME	macula edema		flow-volume
	manic episode	MEG	magnetoencephalogram
	medical events	MEL B	melarsoprol
	medical examiner	MEN	meningeal
	mestranol		meninges
	Methodist		meningitis

	memory	MFAT	multifocal atrial tachycardia
MEN (II)	multiple endocrine neoplasia (type II)	MFB	metallic foreign body
MEO	malignant external otitis	MFD	memory for design
MEOS	microsomal ethanol oxidizing system		midforceps delivery
			milk-free diet
MEP	maximal expiratory pressure	MFEM	maximal forced expiratory maneuver
	meperidine	MFFT	Matching Familiar Figures Test
mEq	milliequivalent		
mEq/24 H	millequivalents per 24 hours	MFH	malignant fibrous histiocytoma
mEq/L	milliequivalents per liter	MFR	mid-forceps rotation
M/E ratio	myeloid/erythroid ratio		myofascial release
MES	mesial	MFT	muscle function test
MET	medical emergency treatment	MFVNS	middle fossa vestibular nerve section
	metabolic	MFVPT	Motor Free Visual Perception Test
	metamyelocytes		
	metastasis	MG	Marcus Gunn
META	metamyelocytes		Michaelis-Gutmann (bodies)
METHb	methemoglobin		
methyl CCNU	semustine		milligram (mg)
			myasthenia gravis
methyl G	mitroguazone dihydrochloride	Mg	magnesium
		μg	microgram (1/1000 of a milligram)
methyl GAG	mitroguazone dihydrochloride		
		mg%	milligrams per 100 milliliters
METS	metabolic equivalents (multiples of resting oxygen uptake)	MGCT	malignant glandular cell tumor
	metastasis	mg/dl	milligrams per 100 milliliters
METT	maximum exercise tolerance test	MGF	macrophage growth factor
			mast cell growth factor
MEV	million electron volts		maternal grandfather
MEX	Mexican	mg/kg	milligram per kilogram
MF	Malassezia folliculitis *Malassezia furfur*	mg/kg/d	milligram per kilogram per day
		mg/kg/hr	milligram per kilogram per hour
	masculinity/femininity		
	meat free	MGM	maternal grandmother
	methotrexate, fluorouracil and calcium leucovorin		milligram (mg is correct)
		MGN	membranous glomerulonephritis
	midcavity forceps		
	mid forceps	MgO	magnesium oxide
	mycosis fungoides	MG/OL	molecular genetics/oncology laboratory
	myocardial fibrosis		
M & F	male and female	MGP	Marcus-Gunn's pupil
	mother and father		

MGS	malignant glandular schwannoma		*Treponema pallidum*
		MHW	medial heel wedge
MgSO₄	magnesium sulfate (Epsom salt)		mental health worker
		MHxR	medical history review
mgtt	minidrop (60 drops = 1 mL)	MHz	megahertz
		MI	membrane intact
MGUS	monoclonal gammopathy of undetermined significance		mental illness
			mental institution
			mitral insufficiency
M-GXT	multi-stage graded exercise test		myocardial infarction
		MIA	medically indigent adult
MH	malignant hyperthermia		missing in action
	marital history	MIBG	meta-iodobenzyl guanidine
	menstrual history		
	mental health	MIC	maternal and infant care
	moist heat		methacholine inhalation challenge
MHA	mental health assistant		
	methotrexate, hydrocortisone, and cytarabine (ARA-C)		medical intensive care
			microscope
			microcytic erythrocytes
	microangiopathic hemolytic anemia		minimum inhibitory concentration
	microhemagglutination	MICA	mentally ill chemical abuser
MHA-TP	microhemagglutination-*Treponema pallidum*		
		MICN	mobile intensive care nurse
MHB	maximum hospital benefit		
	methemoglobin	MICR	methacholine inhalation challenge response
MHBSS	modified Hank's balanced salt solution		
		MICRO	microcytes
MHC	major histocompatibility complex	MICU	medical intensive care unit
			mobile intensive care unit
	mental health center (clinic)	MID	multi-infarct dementia
		Mid I	middle insomnia
	mental health counselor	MID EPIS	midline episiotomy
M/hct	microhematocrit	MIE	maximim inspiratory effort
mHg	millimeters of mercury		
MHI	Mental Health Index (information)		medical improvement expected
MH/MR	mental health and mental retardation	MIF	Merthiolate® iodine-formalin
			migration inhibitory factor
MHN	massive hepatic necrosis	MIFR	mid-inspiratory flow rate
MHRI	Mental Health Research Institute	MIF 50%VC	mid-inspiratory flow at 50% of vital capacity
MHS	major histocompatibility system	MIH	migraine with interparoxysmal headache
	malignant hyperthermia susceptible		
MHTAP	microhemagglutination assay for antibody to	MIL	military
			mother-in-law

MIN	mineral	ML	malignant lymphoma
	minimum		middle lobe
	minor		midline
	minute (min)	mL	milliliter
MINE	mesna uroprotection, ifosfamide, mitoxantrone, and etoposide	M/L	monocyte to lymphocyte (ratio)
			mother-in-law
		MLA	mento-laeva anterior
MINE	medical improvement not expected	MLC	minimal lethal concentration
MIO	minimum identifiable odor		mixed lymphocyte culture
			multilevel care
MIP	maximum inspiratory pressure		multilumen catheter
		MLD	masking level difference
	maximum-intensity projection		metachromatic leukodystrophy
	mean intrathoracic pressure		minimal lethal dose
		MLE	midline (medial) episiotomy
	medical improvement possible	MLF	median longitudinal fasciculus
	metacarpointerphalangeal		
MIRD	medical internal radiation dose	MLNS	mucocutaneous lymph node syndrome
MIRP	myocardial infarction rehabilitation program	MLP	mento-laeva posterior
		MLR	middle latency response
MIS	minimally invasive surgery		mixed lymphocyte reaction
	mitral insufficiency		multiple logistic regression
MISC	miscarriage		
	miscellaneous	MLT	mento-laeva transversa
MISO	misonidazole	MLU	mean length of utterance
MISS	Modified Injury Severity Score (scale)	MM	malignant melanoma
			Marshall-Marchetti
MIT	meconium in trachea		medial malleolus
	miracidia immobilization test		meningococcic meningitis
			mercaptopurine and methotrexate
MITO-C	mitomycin		
mix mon	mixed monitor		methadone maintenance
MJ	marijuana		millimeter (mm)
	megajoule		morbidity and mortality
MJT	Mead Johnson tube		motor meal
μkat	microkatal (micro-moles/sec)		mucous membrane
			multiple myeloma
MKAB	may keep at bedside	mM.	millimole
MKB	married, keeping baby	M&M	milk and molasses
MK-CSF	megakaryocyte colony-stimulating factor		morbidity and mortality
		MMA	methylmalonic acid
MKM	microgram per kilogram per minute		methylmethacrylate
		MMC	mitomycin (mitomycin C)

MMECT	multiple monitor electroconvulsive therapy		Mn	manganese
			M&N	morning and night
			MNC	mononuclear leukocytes
MMEFR	maximal mid-expiratory flow rate		M/NCV	motor nerve conduction velocity
MMF	mean maximum flow		MND	modified neck dissection
MMFR	maximal mid-expiratory flow rate			motor neuron disease (correction)
mmHg	millimeters of mercury		MNF	myelinated nerve fibers
MMK	Marshall-Marchetti-Krantz (cystourethroplexy)		MNG	multinodular goiter
			MNM	mononeuritis multiplex
MMM	mucous membrane moist		MNR	marrow neutrophil reserve
	myelofibrosis with mycloid metaplasia		MNSc	Master of Nursing Science
MMMT	metastatic mixed müllerian tumor		Mn SSEPS	median nerve somatosensory evoked potentials
MMOA	maxillary mandibular odontectomy alveolectomy		MNTB	medial nucleus of the trapezoid body
mmol	millimole		MO	medial oblique (x-ray view)
μmol	micromole			mesio-occlusal
MMPI	Minnesota Multiphasic Personality Inventory			mineral oil
				month (mo)
MMPI-D	Minnesota Multiphasic Personality Inventory-Depression Scale			months old
				morbidly obese
				mother
6-MMPR	6-methylmercaptopurine riboside		Mo	molybdenum
			MOA	mechanism of action
MMR	measles, mumps, and rubella		MoAb	monoclonal antibody
			MOB	medical office building
	midline malignant reticulosis		MOB-PT	mitomycin, vincristine, bleomycin, and cisplatin
MMS	Mini-Mental State (examination)		MOC	Medical Officer on Call
MMT	manual muscle test			mother of child
	Mini Mental Test		MOD	maturity onset diabetes
	mixed müllerian tumors			medical officer of the day
MMTP	Methadone Maintenance Treatment Program			mesio-occlusodistal
				moderate
MMTV	malignant mesothelioma of the tunica vaginalis			multiorgan dysfunction
			MODM	mature-onset diabetes mellitus
	monomorphic ventricular tachycardia		MODY	maturity onset diabetes of youth
MMV	mandatory minute volume		MOE	movement of extremities
MMWR	*Morbidity and Mortality Weekly Report*		MOF	methoxyflurane
MN	midnight			methotrexate, vincristine, and fluorouracil
	mononuclear			

MOFS	multiple-organ failure syndrome
MoICU	mobile intensive care unit
MOJAC	mood orientation, judgement, affect, and content
MOM	milk of magnesia
	mucoid otitis media
MON	monitor
mono.	infectious mononucleosis
	monocyte
	monospot
MOP	medical outpatient
8 MOP	methoxsalen
MOPP	mechlorethamine, vincristine, procarbazine, and prednisone
MOPV	monovalent oral poliovirus vaccine
MOR	morphine
MOS	mirror optical system
	months
mOsm	milliosmole
MOS sf-20	Medical Outcomes Study, short form 20
mOsmol	milliosmole
MOT	motility examination
MOTT	mycobacteria other than tubercle
MOUS	multiple occurrences of unexplained symptoms
MOV	minimum obstructive volume
	multiple oral vitamin
MOW	Meals on Wheels
MP	melphalan and prednisone
	menstrual period
	mercaptopurine
	metacarpal phalangeal joint
	moist park
	mouthpiece
M & P	Millipore and phase
4 MP	methylpyrazole
4MP4	methylpyrazole
6-MP	mercaptopurine
MPA	main pulmonary artery

	medroxyprogesterone acetate
MPa	megapascal
MPAG	McGill Pain Assessment Questionnaire
MPAP	mean pulmonary artery pressure
MPB	male pattern baldness
MPC	mucopurulent cervicitis
MPCN	microscopically positive and culturally negative
MPCU	medical progressive care unit
MPD	maximum permissable dose
	multiple personality disorder
MPE	mean prediction error
MPF	methylparaben free
MPGN	membranoproliferative glomerulonephritis
MPH	Master of Public Health
	methylphenidate
MPI	Maudsley Personality Inventory
MPJ	metacarpophalangeal joint
mpk	milligram per kilogram
MPL	maximum permissable level
MPM	Mortality Prediction Model
MPN	multiple primary neoplasms
MPO	myeloperoxidase
MPOA	medial preoptic area
MPP	massive periretinal proliferation
MPQ	McGill Pain Questionnaire
MPPT	methylprednisolone pulse therapy
MPS	mononuclear phagocyte system
	mucopolysaccharidosis
	multiphasic screening
MPSS	methylprednisolone sodium succinate
MPTRD	motor, pain, touch, reflex, and deficit

MPU	maternal pediatric unit	MRM	modified radical mastectomy
MPV	mean platelet volume		
MQ	memory quotient	MRN	medical resident's note
MR	Maddox rod	mRNA	messenger ribonucleic acid
	magnetic resonance		
	manifest refraction	MRS	magnetic resonance spectroscopy
	may repeat		
	measles-rubella		methicillin-resistant *Staphylococcus aureus*
	medial rectus		
	medical record	MRSA	methicillin-resistant *Staphylococcus aureus*
	mental retardation		
	milliroentgen	MRSE	methicillin-resistant *Staphylococcus epidermidis*
	mitral regurgitation		
	moderate resistance		
M&R	measure and record	MS	mass spectroscopy
MR × 1	may repeat times one (once)		Master of Science
			medical student
MRA	main renal artery		mental status
	medical record administrator		milk shake
			minimal support
	midright atrium		mitral sounds
MRAN	medical resident admitting note		mitral stenosis
			morning stiffness
MRAP	mean right atrial pressure		morphine sulfate
MRAS	main renal artery stenosis		multiple sclerosis
MRC	Master of Rehabilitation Counseling		muscle strength
			musculoskeletal
MRCP	mental retardation, cerebral palsy	M & S	microculture and sensitivity
MRD	margin reflex distance	MS III	third-year medical student
	Medical Records Department	MSAF	meconium-stained amniotic fluid
	minimal residual disease	MSAFP	maternal serum alpha-fetoprotein
MRDD	Mental Retardation and Development Disabilities	MSAP	mean systemic arterial pressure
MRDM	malnutrition-related diabetes mellitus	MSBOS	maximum surgical blood order schedule
MRE	manual resistance exercise	MSCA	McCarthy Scales of Children's Abilities
MRFC	mouse rosette-forming cells	MSCCC	Master Sciences, Certified Clinical Competence
MRG	murmurs, rubs, and gallops	MSCU	medical special care unit
MRH	Maddox rod hyperphoria	MSCWP	musculoskeletal chest wall pain
MRI	magnetic resonance imaging	MSD	microsurgical discectomy
MRL	moderate rubra lochia		mid-sleep disturbance
MRLVD	maximum residue limits of veterinary drugs	MSDS	material safety data sheet
		MSE	Mental Status Examination

Msec	milliseconds	MSTI	multiple soft tissue injuries
MSEL	myasthenic syndrome of Eaton-Lambert	MSU	maple syrup urine
MSER	mean systolic ejection rate		midstream urine
		MSUD	maple-syrup urine disease
	Mental Status Examination Record	MSW	Master of Social Work
MSF	meconium-stained fluid		multiple stab wounds
	megakaryocyte stimulating factor	MT	empty
			macular target
MSG	methysergide		malaria therapy
	monosodium glutamate		malignant teratoma
MSH	melanocyte-stimulating hormone		medical technologist
			metatarsal
MSI	magnetic source imaging		middle turbinate
MSIR®	morphine sulfate immediate release tablets		monitor technician
			muscles and tendons
			music therapy
MSIS	Multiple Severity of Illness System	M/T	masses of tenderness
			myringotomy with tubes
MSK	medullary sponge kidney	M & T	*Monilia* and *Trichomonas*
MSL	midsternal line		myringotomy and tubes
MSLT	multiple sleep latency test	MTAD	tympanic membrane of the left ear
MSM	mid-systolic murmur	MTAS	tympanic membrane of the left ear
MSN	Master of Science in Nursing	MTAU	tympanic membranes of both ears
MSO	mentally stable and oriented	MTB	*Mycobacterium tuberculosis*
	mental status, oriented		
MSO₄	morphine sulfate (this is a dangerous abbreviation)	MTBE	methyl tert-butyl ether
		MTC	magnetization transfer contrast
MSPN	medical student progress notes		medullary thyroid carcinoma
MSPU	medical short procedure unit		mitomycin
MSQ	meters squared	MTD	Monroe tidal drainage
MSR	muscle stretch reflexes	MTDI	maximum tolerable daily intake
MSRPP	Multidimensional Scale for Rating Psychiatric Patients	MTET	modified treadmill exercise testing
MSS	Marital Satisfaction Scale	MTG	mid-thigh girth
	mean sac size	MTI	malignant teratoma intermediate
	minor surgery suite	MTM	modified Thayer-Martin medium
MSSA	methicillin-susceptible *Staphylococcus aureus*		
MSS-CR	mean sac size and crown-rump length	MTP	master treatment plan
			medical termination of pregnancy
MST	mean survival time		
MSTA®	mumps skin test antigen		metatarsal phalangeal

MTR	mother	MVD	microvascular decompression
MTR-O̅	no masses, tenderness, or rebound		mitral valve disease
			multivessel disease
MTRS	Licensed Master Therapeutic Recreation Specialist	MVE	mitral valve (leaflet) excursion
		MVI	multiple vitamin injection
MTST	maximal treadmill stress test	MVI®	trade name for parenteral multivitamins
MTT	methylthiotetrazole	MVI 12®	trade name for parenteral multivitamins
MTU	malignant teratoma undifferentiated	MVO	mixed venous oxygen saturation
	methylthiouracil	MVO₂	myocardial oxygen consumption
MTX	methotrexate		
MTZ	mitoxantrone	MVP	mean venous pressure
MU	million units		mitral valve prolapse
mU	milliunits	MVPP	mechlorethamine, vinblastine, procarbazine, and prednisone
MUA	manipulation under anesthesia		
MUAC	middle upper arm circumference		
MUGA	multiple gated acquisition (scan)	MVR	massive vitreous retraction
			micro-vitreoretinal (blade)
MUGX	multiple gated acquisition exercise		mitral valve regurgitation
			mitral valve replacement
mus-lig	musculoligamentous	MVS	mitral valve stenosis
MuLV	murine leukemia virus		motor, vascular, and sensory
MUU	mouse uterine units		
MV	mechanical ventilation	MVV	maximum voluntary ventilation
	millivolts		
	minute volume		mixed vespid venom
	mitoxantrone and etoposide	MWD	microwave diathermy
		MWI	Medical Walk-In (Clinic)
	mitral valve	MWS	Mickety-Wilson syndrome
	mixed venous	MWT	malpositioned wisdom teeth
	multivesicular		
MVA	malignant vertricular arrhythmias	Mx	myringotomy
		My	myopia
	mitral valve area	myelo	myelocytes
	motor vehicle accident		myelogram
M-VAC	methotrexate, vinblastine, doxorubicin, and cisplatin	MYD	mydriatic
		MyG	myasthenia gravis
		MYR	myringotomy
MVAC	methotrexate, vinblastine, doxorubicin, and cisplatin	MYS	medium yellow soft (stools)
		MZ	monozygotic
MVB	mixed venous blood	MZL	marginal zone lymphocyte
MVC	maximal voluntary contraction	MZT	monozygotic twins

113

N

N negative
 Negro
 nerve
 never
 newton
 nipple
 no
 nodes
 normal
 not
 noun
 NPH insulin
 size of sample
N_2 nitrogen
5'-N 5'-nucleotidase
Na sodium
NA Narcotics Anonymous
 Native American
 Negro adult
 nicotinic acid
 normal axis
 not admitted
 not applicable
 not available
 nurse aide
 Nurse Anesthetist
 nursing assistant
N & A normal and active
NAA neutron activation
  analysis
 no apparent abnormalities
NAAC no apparent anesthesia
  (anesthetic)
  complications
NAATPT not available at the
  present time
NAB not at bedside
NABS normoactive bowel
  sounds
NAC acetylcysteine
  (N-acetylcysteine)
NaClO sodium hypochlorite
NaCl sodium chloride (salt)
NAD nicotinamide adenine
  dinucleotide

 no active disease
 no acute distress
 no apparent distress
 no appreciable disease
 normal axis deviation
 nothing abnormal detected
NADPH nicotinamide adenine
  dinucleotide phosphate
NADSIC no apparent disease seen
  in chest
NaF sodium fluoride
NAF nafcillin
 Negro adult female
NAG narrow angle glaucoma
$NaHCO_3$ sodium bicarbonate
NAI no acute inflammation
 non-accidental injury
NaI sodium iodide
NAION non-arteritic ischemic
  optic neuropathy
NANB non-A, non-B (hepatitis)
NANBH non-A, non-B hepatitis
NANDA North American Nursing
  Diagnosis Association
NAP narrative, assessment, and
  plan
NAPA N-acetyl procainamide
NAPD no active pulmonary
  disease
Na Pent Pentothal Sodium®
NAR no adverse reaction
 not at risk
NARC narcotic(s)
NAS nasal
 neonatal abstinence
  syndrome
 no added salt
NAT N-acetyltransferase
 no action taken
 non-accidental trauma
$Na^{99m}TcO_4^-$ sodium pertechnetate
  Tc 99m
NAW nasal antral window
NB nail bed
 needle biopsy
 newborn
 nitrogen balance
 note well
NBC non-bed care

NBD	neurologic bladder dysfunction	NCB	natural childbirth
	no brain damage		no code blue
NBF	not breast fed	NCC	no concentrated carbohydrates
NBH	new bag (bottle) hung	NCD	normal childhood diseases
NBHH	newborn helpful hints		not considered disabling
NBI	no bone injury	NCE	new chemical entity
NBICU	newborn intensive care unit	NCEP	National Cholesterol Education Program
NBM	no bowel movement	NCF	neutrophilic chemotactic factor
	normal bone marrow		
	normal bowel movement	NCI	National Cancer Institute
	nothing by mouth	NCJ	needle catheter jejunostomy
NBN	newborn nursery		
NBP	needle biopsy of prostate	NCL	neuronal ceroid lipofuscinosis
NBQC	narrow base quad cane		
NBR	no blood return		nuclear cardiology laboratory
NBS	newborn screen (serum thyroxine and phenylketonuria)	NCM	nailfold capillary microscope
	no bacteria seen	NCNC	normochromic, normocytic
	normal bowel sound		
NBT	nitroblue tetrazolium reduction (tests)	NCO	no complaints offered
			non-commissioned officer
NBTE	nonbacterial thrombotic endocarditis	NCP	nursing care plan
		NCPAP	nasal continuous positive airway pressure
NBTNF	newborn, term, normal female		
		NCPR	no cardiopulmonary resuscitation
NBTNM	newborn, term, normal, male	NCRC	non–child-resistant container
NC	nasal cannula		
	Negro child	NCS	nerve conduction studies
	neurologic check		no concentrated sweets
	no change		zinostatin (neocarzinostatin)
	no charge		
	no complaints	NCT	neutron capture therapy
	noncontributory		noncontact tonometry
	nose clamp	NCV	nerve conduction velocity
	nose clips		nuclear venogram
	not completed	ND	nasal deformity
	not cultured		natural death
NCA	neurocirculatory asthenia		neck dissection
	no congenital abnormalities		neonatal death
			neurological development
N/CAN	nasal cannula		no disease
NCAP	nasal continuous airway pressure		nondisabling
			non-distended
NCAS	neocarzinostatin		none detectable
NC/AT	normocephalic atraumatic		normal delivery

	normal development	NEFG	normal external female genitalia
	nose drops		
	not diagnosed	NEF	negative expiratory force
	not done	NEFA	non-esterified fatty acids
	nothing done	NEG	negative
	Nursing Doctorate		neglect
N&D	nodular and diffuse	NEPHRO	nephrogram
Nd	neodymium	NEM	no evidence of malignancy
NDA	New Drug Application		
	no data available	NEMD	nonspecific esophageal motility disorder
	no detectable activity		
NDD	no dialysis days	NEOH	neonatal high risk
NDF	neutral density filter (test)	NEOM	neonatal medium risk
	no disease found	NEP	no evidence of pathology
NDI	neurogenic diabetes insipidus	NER	no evidence of recurrence
		NERD	no evidence of recurrent disease
Nd/NT	nondistended, nontender		
NDP	net dietary protein	NES	not elsewhere specified
NDR	neurotic depressive reaction	NET	naso-endotracheal tube
		NETA	norethisterone acetate
	normal detrusor reflex	NETT	nasal endotracheal tube
NDS	Neurologic Disability Score	NEX	nose to ear to xiphoid
			number of acquisitions or excitations
NDST	neurodevelopmental screening test		
		NF	Negro female
NDT	neurodevelopmental treatment		neurofibromatosis
			none found
	noise detection threshold		not found
NDV	Newcastle disease virus		nursed fair
Nd:YAG	neodymium:yttrium-aluminum-garnet (laser)	NFD	no family doctor
		NFL	nerve fiber layer
NE	neurological examination	NFLX	norfloxacin
	never exposed	NFP	no family physician
	no effect	NFTD	normal full-term delivery
	no enlargement	NFTSD	normal full-term spontaneous delivery
	norethindrone		
	norepinephrine	NFTT	nonorganic failure to thrive
	not elevated		
	not examined	NFW	nursed fairly well
NEAC	norethindrone acetate	NG	nanogram
NEB	hand-held nebulizer		nasogastric
NEC	necrotizing entercolitis		nitroglycerin
	noise equivalent counts		no growth
	not elsewhere classified	NGB	neurogenic bladder
NED	no evidence of disease	NGF	nerve growth factor
NEEG	normal electroencephalo-gram	n giv	not given
		NGR	nasogastric replacement
NEEP	negative end-expiratory pressure	NGRI	not guilty by reason of insanity

NGT	nasogastric tube
	normal glucose tolerance
NGU	nongonococcal urethritis
NH	nursing home
NHC	neighborhood health center
	neonatal hypocalcemia
	nursing home care
NHCU	nursing home care unit
NH_3	ammonia
NH_4Cl	ammonium chloride
NHCU	nursing home care unit
NHD	normal hair distribution
NHL	nodular histiocytic lymphoma
	non-Hodgkin's lymphomas
nHL	normalized hearing level
NHP	Nottingham Health Profile
	nursing home placement
NI	neurological improvement
	no improvement
	no information
	none indicated
	not identified
	not isolated
NIA	no information available
NIAID	National Institute of Allergy and Infectious Diseases
NIAL	not in active labor
NICC	neonatal intensive care center
NICHD	National Institute of Child Health and Human Development
NICS	non-invasive carotid studies
NICU	neonatal intensive care unit
	neurosurgical intensive care unit
NID	not in distress
NIDD	non–insulin-dependent diabetes
NIDDM	non–insulin-dependent diabetes mellitus
NIF	negative inspiratory force
	not in file
NIFS	non-invasive flow studies

NIG	NSAIA (non-steroidal anti-inflamatory agent) induced gastropathy
NIH	National Institutes of Health
NIHL	noise-induced hearing loss
NIL	not in labor
NIMAs	non-inherited maternal antigens
NIMHDIS	National Institute for Mental Health Diagnostic Interview Schedule
NINU	neuro intermediate nursing unit
NINVS	non-invasive neurovascular studies
NIP	no infection present
	no inflammation present
NIPAs	non-inherited paternal antigens
Nitro	nitroglycerin (this is a dangerous abbreviation)
	sodium nitroprusside
NIVLS	non-invasive vascular laboratory studies
NJ	nasojejunal
NK	natural killer (cells)
	not known
NKA	no known allergies
nkat	nanokatal (nanomole/sec)
NKB	no known basis
NKC	nonketotic coma
NKDA	no known drug allergies
NKFA	no known food allergies
NKHA	nonketotic hyperosmolar acidosis
NKHS	nonketotic hyperosmolar syndrome
NKMA	no known medication allergies
NL	nasolacrimal
	normal
NLB	needle liver biopsy
NLC & C	normal libido, coitus, and climax
NLD	nasolacrimal duct
	necrobiosis lipoidica diabeticorum

NLE	neonatal lupus erythematosus	NMSIDS	near-miss sudden infant death syndrome
	nursing late entry	NMT	nebulized mist treatment
NLF	nasolabial fold		no more than
NLFGNR	non-lactose fermenting gram-negative rod	NMTB	neuromuscular transmission blockade
NLP	no light perception	NMT(R)	Nuclear Medicine Technologist Registered
	nodular liquifying panniculitis	NN	narrative notes
NLS	neonatal lupus syndrome		neonatal
NLT	not later than		normal nursery
	not less than		nurses' notes
NM	Negro male	N/N	negative/negative
	neuromuscular	NNBC	node-negative breast cancer
	nodular melanoma		
	nonmalignant	NND	neonatal death
	not measurable	NNE	neonatal necrotizing enterocolitis
	not measured		
	not mentioned	NNM	Nicolle-Novy-MacNeal (media)
	nuclear medicine		
	nurse manager	NNL	no new laboratory (test orders)
N & M	nerves and muscles		
	night and morning	NNN	normal newborn nursery
NMBA	neuromuscular blocking agent	NNO	no new orders
		NNP	Neonatal Nurse Practitioner
NMD	Normosol M and 5% Dextrose®		
		N:NPK	grams of nitrogen to non-protein kilocalories
NMI	no manifest improvement		
	no mental illness	NNS	neonatal screen (hematocrit, total bilirubin, and total protein)
	no middle initial		
	normal male infant		
NMKB	not married, keeping baby		
NMN	no middle name	NNT	number needed to treat
NMNKB	not married, not keeping baby	NNU	net nitrogen utilization
		NO	nasal oxygen
nmol	nanomole		nitroglycerin ointment
NMP	normal menstrual period		nitrous oxide
NMR	nuclear magnetic resonance (same as magnetic resonance imaging)		none obtained
			nonobese
			number (no.)
			nursing office
NMRT (R)	Nuclear Medicine Radiologic Technologist (Registered)	N_2O	nitrous oxide
		$N_2O:O_2$	nitrous oxide to oxygen ratio
		noc.	night
NMS	neuroleptic malignant syndrome	noct	nocturnal
		NOD	nonobese diabetic
NMSE	normalized mean square root		notify of death
		NOK	next of kin

NOL	not on label	NPDL	nodular poorly differentiated lymphocytic
NOM	nonsuppurative otitis media		
NOMI	nonocclusive mesenteric infarction	NPDR	nonproliferative diabetic retinopathy
NONMEM	non-linear mixed-effects model	NPE	neuropsychologic examination
non pal	not palpable		no palpable enlargement
NOOB	not out of bed		normal pelvic examination
NOR	norethynodrel		
	normal	NPEM	nocturnal penile erection monitoring
	nortriptyline		
NOR-EPI	norepinephrine	NPF	nasopharyngeal fiberscope
norm	normal		no predisposing factor
NOS	not on staff	NPH	a type of insulin (isophane)
	not otherwise specified		
NOSIE	Nurse's Observation Scale (Schedule) for Inpatient Evaluation		no previous history
			normal pressure hydrocephalus
NOT	nocturnal oxygen therapy	NPG	nonpregnant
NOU	not on unit	NPhx	nasopharynx
NP	nasal prongs	NPI	no present illness
	nasopharyngeal	NPJT	nonparoxysmal junctional tachycardia
	near point		
	neurophysin	NPK	non-protein kilocalories
	neuropsychiatric	NPN	nonprotein nitrogen
	newly presented	NPO	nothing by mouth
	nonpalpable	NPOD	Neuropsychiatric Officer of the Day
	no pain		
	not performed	NPP	normal postpartum
	not pregnant	NPPNG	nonpenicillinase-producing *Neisseria gonorrhoeae*
	not present		
	nursed poorly		
	nuclear pharmacist	NPR	normal pulse rate
	nuclear pharmacy		nothing per rectum
	nurse practitioner	NPSA	nonphysician surgical assistant
NPA	nasal pharyngeal airway		
	near point of accommodation	NPT	nocturnal penile tumescence
			normal pressure and temperature
	no previous admission		
NPAT	nonparoxysmal atrial tachycardia	NPU	net protein utilization
		NPV	nothing per vagina
NPC	near point convergences	NQMI	non-Q wave myocardial infarction
	nodal premature contractions		
	nonpatient contact	NR	do not repeat
	nonproductive cough		no refills
	nonprotein calorie		no report
NPD	no pathological diagnosis		no response

	no return		not seen
	nonreactive		not significant
	nonrebreathing		nursing service
	normal range		nylon suture
	normal reaction	NSA	no salt added
	not reached		no significant abnormality
	not reacting		normal serum albumin
NRAF	non-rheumatic atrial fibrillation	NSABP	National Surgical Adjuvant Breast Project
NRB	non-rebreather	NSAD	no signs of acute disease
NRBC	normal red blood cell nucleated red blood cell	NSAIA	non-steroidal anti-inflammatory agent
NRBS	non-rebreathing system	NSAID	non-steroidal anti-inflammatory drug
NRC	National Research Council	NSBGP	non-specific bowel gas pattern
	normal retinal correspondence	NSC	no significant change nonservice-connected
	Nuclear Regulatory Commission	NSCD	nonservice-connected disability
NREM	nonrapid eye movement	NSCFPT	no significant change from previous tracing
NREMS	nonrapid eye movement sleep	NSCLC	non–small-cell lung cancer
NRF	normal renal function	NSCST	nipple stimulation contraction stress test
NRI	nerve root involvement		
	nerve root irritation	NSD	nasal septal deviation
	no recent illnesses		no significant disease (difference, defect, deviation)
NRM	non rebreathing mask		
	no regular medicines		
	normal range of motion		nominal standard dose
	normal retinal movement		normal spontaneous delivery
NRN	no return necessary		
NRO	neurology	NSDA	non-steroid dependent asthmatic
NROM	normal range of motion		
NRP	non-reassuring patterns	NSDU	neonatal stepdown unit
NRPR	non-breathing pressure relieving	NSE	neuron-specific enolase normal saline enema (0.9% sodium chloride)
NRT	neuromuscular reeducation techniques		
		N s̄ E	nausea without emesis
NS	nephrotic syndrome	NSFTD	normal spontaneous full-term delivery
	neurological signs		
	neurosurgery	NSG	nursing
	nipple stimulation	NSGCT	nonseminomatous germ cell tumors
	nodular sclerosis		
	no-show	NSHD	nodular sclerosing Hodgkin's disease
	nonsmoker		
	normal saline solution (0.9% sodium chloride solution)	NSI	negative self-image
			no signs of infection
	no sample		

	no signs of inflammation		normal temperature
NSICU	neurosurgery intensive care unit	.	nortriptyline
			not tender
NSILA	nonsuppressible insulin-like activity		not tested
			nourishment taken
NSN	nephrotoxic serum nephritis		nursing technician
		N&T	nose and throat
NSO	Neosporin® ointment	NTBR	not to be resuscitated
NSP	neck and shoulder pain	NTC	neurotrauma center
NSPVT	nonsustained polymorphic ventricular tachycardia	NTD	neural tube defects
		NTE	not to exceed
NSR	nasoseptal repair	NTF	normal throat flora
	nonspecific reaction	NTG	nitroglycerin
	normal sinus rhythm		nontoxic goiter
	not seen regularly		nontreatment group
NSS	neurological signs stable	NTGO	nitroglycerin ointment
	normal size and shape	NTL	nortriptyline
	not statistically significant	NTM	nocturnal tumescence monitor
	nutritional support service		
	sodium chloride 0.9% (normal saline solution)	NTMB	nontuberculous myobacteria
1/2 NSS	sodium chloride 0.45% (1/2 normal saline solution)	NTMI	non-transmural myocardial infarction
		NTND	not tender, not distended
NSSL	normal size, shape, and location	NTP	Nitropaste® (nitroglycerin ointment)
NSSP	normal size, shape, and position		normal temperature and pressure
			sodium nitroprusside
NSSTT	nonspecific ST and T (wave)	NTS	nasotracheal suction
NSST-TWCs	nonspecific ST-T wave changes		nucleus tractus solitarii
		NTT	nasotracheal tube
NST	non-stress test	NTU	nephelometric turbidity units
	not sooner than		
	nutritional support team	NU	name unknown
NSTD	non-sexually transmitted disease	NUD	nonulcer dyspepsia
		NUG	necrotizing ulcerative gingivitis
NSTT	nonseminomatous testicular tumors		
		nullip	nullipara
NSU	neurosurgical unit	NV	nausea and vomiting
	nonspecific urethritis		near vision
NSV	nonspecific vaginitis		neurovascular
NSVD	normal spontaneous vaginal delivery		next visit
			nonvaccinated
NSVT	non-sustained ventricular tachycardia		nonvenereal
			nonveteran
NSX	neurosurgical examination		normal value
NSY	nursery		not verified
NT	nasotracheal	N&V	nausea and vomiting

NVA	near visual acuity		obvious
NVAF	nonvalvular atrial fibrillation		occlusal
			often
NVD	nausea, vomiting, and diarrhea		open
			oral
	neck vein distention		ortho
	neovascularization of the disc		other
			oxygen
	neurovesicle dysfunction		pint
	no venereal disease		zero
	nonvalvular disease	ō	negative
NVDC	nausea, vomiting, diarrhea, and constipation		none
			pint
			without
NVE	native	$_1O_2$	singlet oxygen
	native valve endocarditis	O_2	both eyes
	neovascularization elsewhere		oxygen
NVG	neovascular glaucoma	O_2	superoxide
	neoviridogrisein	OA	occiput anterior
NVL	neurovascular laboratory		on arrival
NVS	neurological vital signs		ophthalmic artery
NVSS	normal variant short stature		oral airway
			oral alimentation
NW	naked weight		osteoarthritis
	nasal wash		Overeaters Anonymous
	not weighed	O & A	observation and assessment
NWB	non-weight bearing		odontectomy and alveoloplasty
NWC	number of words chosen		
NWD	neuroleptic withdrawal	OAC	oral anticoagulant(s)
	normal well developed		overaction
Nx	nephrectomy	OAD	obstructive airway disease
NYD	not yet diagnosed		occlusive arterial disease
NYHA	New York Heart Association (classification of heart disease)	OAE	otoacoustic emissions
		OAF	oral anal fistula
			osteoclast activating factor
		OAG	open angle glaucoma
nyst	nystagmus	OAP	old age pension
NZ	enzyme	OASDHI	Old Age, Survivors, Disability, and Health Insurance
		OAS	organic anxiety syndrome
		OASO	overactive superior oblique
	O	OASR	overactive superior rectus
		OAW	oral airway
O	eye	OB	obese
	objective findings		obstetrics

	occult blood	OCNS	Obsessive-Compulsive Neurosis Scale
	osteoblast		
OB-A	obstetrics-aborted	OCP	oral contraceptive pills
OB-Del	obstetrics-delivered		ova, cysts, parasites
OBE-CALP	placebo capsule or tablet	OCS	Obsessive-Compulsive Scale
OBG	obstetrics and gynecology	11-OCS	11-oxycorticosteroid
Ob-Gyn	obstetrics and gynecology	OCT	ornithine carbamyl transferase
Obj	objective		oxytocin challenge test
obl	oblique	OCU	observation care unit
OB-ND	obstetrics-not delivered	OCVM	occult cerebrovascular malformations
OBRR	obstetric recovery room		
OBS	obstetrical service	OD	doctor of optometry
	organic brain syndrome		Officer-of-the-Day
OBT	obtained		once daily (this is a dangerous abbreviation as it is read as right eye)
OC	obstetrical conjugate		
	office call		
	on call		
	only child		on duty
	oral care		optic disc
	oral contraceptive		outdoor
	osteocalcin		overdose
	osteoclast		right eye
O & C	onset and course	Δ OD 450	deviation of optical density at 450
OCA	oculocutaneous albinism		
	open care area	ODA	occipitodextra anterior
	oral contraceptive agent		osmotic driving agent
OCAD	occlusive carotid artery disease	ODAC	on demand analgesia computer
OCC	occlusal	ODAT	one day at a time
OCCC	open chest cardiac compression	ODC	ornithine decarboxylase
			outpatient diagnostic center
occl	occlusion	ODCH	ordinary diseases of childhood
OCCM	open chest cardiac massage		
		ODed	overdosed
OCC PR	open-chest cardiopulmonary resuscitation	ODM	ophthalmodynamometry
		ODN	optokinetic nystagmus
OCC Th	occupational therapy	ODP	occipitodextra transverse
Occup Rx	occupational therapy		offspring of diabetic parents
OCD	obsessive-compulsive disorder		
	osteochondritis dissecans	ODSU	oncology day stay unit
OCG	oral cholecystogram	OE	on examination
OCI	Obsessive-Compulsive Inventory		orthopedic examination
			otitis externa
OCL®	oral colonic lavage	O&E	observation and examination
OCN	Oncology Certified Nurse		
	obsessive compulsive neurosis	OEC	outer ear canal

OER	oxygen enhancement ratios		open heart surgery
OET	oral esophageal tube	OI	opportunistic infection
OETT	oral endotracheal tube		osteogenesis imperfecta
OF	occipital-frontal		otitis interna
	optic fundi	OIF	oil-immersion field
OFC	occipital-frontal circumference	OIH	orthoiodohippurate
	orbitofacial cleft	OIHA	orthoiodohippuric acid
OFLX	ofloxacin	OIU	optical internal urethrotomy
OFM	open face mask	OJ	orange juice (this is a dangerous abbreviation)
OG	Obstetrics-Gynecology orogastric (feeding)		orthoplast jacket
OGT	orogastric tube	OK	all right
OGTT	oral glucose tolerance test		approved
OH	occupational history		correct
	on hand	OKAN	optokinetic after nystagmus
	open heart		
	oral hygiene	OKN	optokinetic nystagmus
	orthostatic hypotension	OL	left eye
	outside hospital		open label (study)
17-OH	17-hydroxycorticosteroids	OLA	occiput left anterior
OHA	oral hypoglycemic agents	OLM	ocular larva migrans
OHC	outer hair cell (in cochlea)	OLP	occipitolaevoanterior
OH Cbl	hydroxycobalamine	OLR	otology, laryngology, and rhinology
17-OHCS	17-hydroxycorticosteroids	OLT	occipitolaevoposterior
OHD	hydroxy vitamin D		orthotopic liver transplantation
	organic heart disease		
OHF	Omsk hemorrhagic fever	OLTx	orthotopic liver transplantation
	overhead frame		
OHFT	overhead frame and trapeze	OM	every morning (this is a dangerous abbreviation)
OHG	oral hypoglycemic		obtuse marginal
OHI	oral hygiene instructions		oral motor
OHIAA	hydroxyindolacetic acid		osteomalacia
OHL	oral hairy leukoplakia		osteomyelitis
OHNS	Otolaryngology, Head, and Neck Surgery (Dept.)		otitis media
		OMA	older maternal age
		OMAS	otitis media, acute, suppurating
OHP	oxygen under hyperbaric pressure	OMCA	otitis media, catarrhalis, acute
OHRP	open heart rehabilitation program	OMCC	otitis media, catarrhalis, chronic
OHRR	open heart recovery room	OME	Office of Medical Examiner
OHS	occupational health service		otitis media with effusion
		7-OMEN	menogaril
	ocular hypoperfusion syndrome	OMFS	oral and maxillofacial surgery

OMI	old myocardial infarct		otorhinolaryngology, and head and neck surgery
OMPA	otitis media, purulent, acute		
OMPC	otitis media, purulent, chronic	OOI	out of isolette
		OOL	onset of labor
OMR	operative mortality rate	OOLR	ophthalmology, otology, laryngology, and rhinology
OMS	oral morphine sulfate organic mental syndrome organic mood syndrome		
		OOP	out of pelvis out of plaster out on pass
OMSA	otitis media secretory (or suppurative) acute		
		OOPS	out of program status
OMSC	otitis media secretory (or suppurative) chronic	OOR	out of room
		OORW	out of radiant warmer
OMVC	open mitral valve commissurotomy	OOS	out of stock
		OOT	out of town
OMVI	operating motor vehicle intoxicated	OOW	out of wedlock
		OP	oblique presentation occiput posterior open operation oropharynx oscillatory potentials osteoporosis outpatient
ON	every night (this is a dangerous abbreviation) optic nerve optic neurophathy oronasal Ortho-Novum® overnight		
		O&P	ova and parasites
		OPA	outpatient anesthesia oral pharyngeal airway
ONC	over-the-needle catheter vincristine (Oncovin®)		
OND	ondansetron	OPB	outpatient basis
ONH	optic nerve head optic nerve hypoplasia	OPC	outpatient catheterization outpatient clinic
		OPCA	olivopontocerebellar atrophy
ONSD	optic nerve sheath decompression		
		op cit	in the work cited
ONSF	optic nerve sheath fenestration	OPD	outpatient department
		O'p'-DDD	mitotane
ONTR	orders not to resuscitate	OPE	outpatient evaluation
OO	ophthalmic ointment oral order other out of	OPG	ocular plethysmography
		OPM	occult primary malignancy
o/o	on account of	OPO	organ procurement organizations
OOB	out of bed		
OOBL	out of bili light	OPOC	oral pharynx, oral cavity
OOBBRP	out of bed with bathroom privileges	OPP	opposite
		OPPG	oculopneumoplethysmography
OOC	onset of contractions out of cast out of control		
		OPS	operations outpatient surgery
OO Con	out of control		
OOD	outer orbital diameter	OPT	optimum
OOH&NS	ophthalmology,		

	outpatient treatment	OSAS	obstructive sleep apnea syndrome
OPT c̄ CA	Ohio pediatric tent with compressed air	OSD	overside drainage
OPT c̄ O₂	Ohio pediatric tent with oxygen	OSFT	outstretched fingertips
		OSHA	Occupational Safety & Health Administration
OPT-NSC	outpatient treatment, non-service connected	OSM S	osmolarity serum
OPT-SC	outpatient treatment, service-connected	OSM U	osmolarity urine
		OSN	off service note
OPV	oral polio vaccine	OSP	outside pass
OR	odd-ratio	OSS	osseous
	oil retention		over-shoulder strap
	open reduction	OT	occiput transverse
	operating room		occupational therapy
	Orthodox		old tuberculin
ORA	occiput right anterior		oxytocin
ORCH	orchiectomy	OTA	open to air
ORIF	open reduction internal fixation	OTC	ornithine transcarbamoy-lase
ORL	otorhinolaryngology		over the counter (sold without prescription)
ORN	operating room nurse		
OROS	ostomotic release oral system	OTD	organ tolerance dose
			out the door
ORP	occiput right posterior	OTH	other
ORS	oral rehydration salts	OTHS	occupational therapy home service
ORT	operating room technician		
	oral rehydration therapy	OTO	otology
	Registered Occupational Therapist	OTR	Occupational Therapist, Registered
OR X1	oriented to time	OT/RT	occupational therapy/recreational therapy
OR X2	oriented to time and place		
OR X3	oriented to time, place, and person		
		OTS	orotracheal suction
OR X4	oriented to person, place, time, and objects (watch, pen, book)	OTT	orotracheal tube
		OU	both eyes
		OURQ	outer upper right quadrant
OS	left eye	OV	office visit
	mouth (this is a dangerous abbreviation as it is read as left eye)		ovary
			ovum
		OVAL	ovalocytes
	occipitosacral	OVF	Octopus® visual field
	opening snap	OVR	Office of Vocational Rehabilitation
	ophthalmic solution (this is a dangerous abbreviation as it is read as left eye)		
		OW	once weekly (this is a dangerous abbreviation)
			outer wall
	oral surgery		out of wedlock
	osmium	O/W	otherwise
OSA	obstructive sleep apnea	OWNK	out of wedlock not keeping

126

				aortic second heart sound
OX	oximeter		PAB	premature atrial beat
Oxi	oximeter (oximetry)			pulmonary artery banding
OXM	pulse oximeter		PAC	cisplatin (Platinol®), doxorubicin (Adriamycin®), and cylcophosphamide
Oxy-5®	benzoyl peroxide			
OXZ	oxazepam			
oz	ounce			
				Physician Assistant, Certified

P

				Port-a-cath®
				premature atrial contraction
P	para			pulmonary artery catheter
	peripheral		PACH	pipers to after coming head
	phosphorus			
	pint		PACO₂	partial pressure (tension) of carbon dioxide, alveolar
	plan			
	protein			
	pulse		PaCO₂	partial pressure (tension) of carbon dioxide, artery
	pupil			
p̄	after			
/P	partial lower denture		PACT	prism and alternate cover test
P/	partial upper denture			
P₂	pulmonic second heart sound		PAC-V	cisplatin, doxorubicin, and cyclophosphamide
P20	Ocusert® P20			
P40	Ocusert® P40		PACU	postanesthesia care unit
³²P	radioactive phosphorus		PAD	peripheral artery disease
PA	paranoid			preliminary anatomic diagnosis
	periapical (x-ray)			
	pernicious anemia			primary affective disorder
	phenol alcohol		PADP	pulmonary arterial diastolic (pressure)
	Physician Assistant			
	pineapple			pulmonary artery diastolic pressure
	posterior-anterior (x-ray)			
	presents again		PAE	postanoxic encephalopathy
	professional association			
	psychiatric aide			postantibiotic effect
	psychoanalysis			progressive assistive exercise
	pulmonary artery			
Pa	pascal		PAEDP	pulmonary artery and end-diastole pressure
P&A	percussion and auscultation			
			PAF	paroxysmal atrial fibrillation
	position and alignment			
				platelet activating factor
P₂>A₂	pulmonic second heart sound greater than		PA&F	percussion, auscultation, and fremitus
			PAGA	premature appropriate for gestational age

PAGE	polyacrylamide gel electrophoresis		pulmonary stenosis
		PAPVC	partial anomalous pulmonary venous connection
PAH	para-aminohippurate phenylalanine hydroxylase pulmonary arterial hypertension		
		PAR	parafin parallel perennial allergic rhinitis platelet aggregate ratio postanesthetic recovery procedures, alternatives, and risks pulmonary arteriolar resistance
PAI	plasminogen activator inhibitor platelet accumulation index		
PAIVS	pulmonary atresia with intact ventricle septum		
PAL	posteroanterior and lateral posterior axillary line	PARA	number of pregnancies
		para	paraplegic
Pa Line	pulmonary artery line	PARC	perennial allergic rhinoconjunctivitis
PALN	para-aortic lymph node		
PALS	pediatric advanced life support	PAROM	passive assistance range of motion
PAM	penicillin aluminum monostearate primary amebic meningoencephalitis	PARR	postanesthesia recovery room
		PARS	postanesthesia recovery score
2-PAM	pralidoxime	PARU	postanesthetic recovery unit
PAMP	pulmonary arterial (artery) mean pressure	PAS	aminosalicylic acid (para-aminosalicylic periodic acid-Schiff (reagent) peripheral anterior synechia pneumatic antiembolic stocking postanesthesia score premature auricular systole Professional Activities Study pulmonary artery stenosis pulsatile antiembolism system (stockings)
PAN	pancuronium periodic alternating nystagmus polyacylonitrile polyarteritis nodosa		
PANESS	physical and neurological examination for soft signs		
PAO_2	alveolar oxygen pressure (tension)		
PaO_2	arterial oxygen pressure (tension)		
PAO	peak acid output		
PAOP	pulmonary artery occlusion pressure	PASA	aminosalicylic acid (para-aminosalicylic acid)
PAP	passive aggressive personality peroxidase-anti-peroxidase primary atypical pneumonia prostatic acid phosphatase pulmonary artery pressure	Pas Ex	passive exercise
		PASG	pneumatic antishock garment
		PASP	pulmonary artery systolic pressure
Pap smear	Papanicolaou smear	PAT	paroxysmal atrial tachycardia
PA/PS	pulmonary atresia/		

	patella	PBMC	peripheral blood
	patient		mononuclear cell
	percent acceleration time	PBMNC	peripheral blood
	platelet aggregation test		mononuclear cell
	preadmission testing	PBN	polymyxin B sulfate,
	pregnancy at term		bacitracin, and
Path.	pathology		neomycin
PAV	Pavulon®	PBO	placebo
PAVM	pulmonary arteriovenous	PBPI	penile-brachial pulse
	malformation		index
PAWP	pulmonary artery wedge	PBS	phosphate-buffered saline
	pressure	PBSC	peripheral blood stem
PAX	periapical x-ray		cells
PB	barometric pressure	PBT₄	protein-bound thyroxine
	parafin bath	PBV	percutaneous balloon
	power building		valvuloplasty
	powder board	PBZ	phenoxybenzamine
	premature beat		phenylbutazone
	Presbyterian		pyribenzamine
	protein-bound	ΦBZ	phenylbutazone
	pudendal block	PC	after meals
Pb	lead		packed cells
	phenobarbital		platelet concentrate
p/b	post-burn		poor condition
P&B	pain and burning		popliteal cyst
	phenobarbital and		posterior chamber
	belladonna		present complaint
PBA	percutaneous bladder		productive cough
	aspiration		professional corporation
PBAL	protected bronchoalveolar		psychiatric counselor
	lavage	PCA	passive cutaneous
PbB	whole blood lead		anaphylaxis
PBC	point of basal convergence		patient care assistant
	pre-bed care		(aide)
	primary biliary cirrhosis		patient controlled
PBD	percutaneous biliary		analgesia
	drainage		porous coated anatomic
	proliferative breast		(joint replacement)
	disease		post ciliary artery
PBE	partial breech extraction		postconceptional age
PBF	placental blood flow		posterior cerebral artery
	pulmonary blood flow		posterior communicating
PBG	porphobilinogen		artery
PBI	protein-bound iodine		procainamide
PBK	pseudophakic bullous		procoagulation activity
	keratopathy	PCB	pancuronium bromide
PBL	peripheral blood		para cervical block
	lymphocyte		prepared childbirth

PCBs	polychlorinated biphenyls	PCOD	polycystic ovarian disease
PCC	pheochromocytoma poison control center	P COMM A	posterior communicating artery
PCCC	pediatric critical care center	PCOS	polycystic ovary syndrome
PCCU	postcoronary care unit	PCP	patient care plan
PCD	postmortem cesarean delivery		phencyclidine *Pneumocystis carinii*
PCE	physical capacities evaluation		pneumonia primary care person
	potentially compensable event		primary care physician pulmonary capillary
PCE®	erythromycin particles in tablets	PCR	pressure polymerase chain reaction
PCEA	patient-controlled epidural analgesia	PCS	protein catabolic rate patient care system
PCFT	platelet complement fixation test		portable cervical spine portacaval shunt
PCG	phonocardiogram		postconcussion syndrome
PCGG	percutaneous coagulation of gasserian ganglion	P c/s PCT	primary cesarean section porphyria cutanea tarda
PCH	paroxysmal cold hemoglobinuria		post coital test posterior chest tube
PC&HS	after meals and at bedtime		progestin challenge test
PCI	prophylactic cranial irradiation	PCU	palliative care unit primary care unit
PCIOL	posterior chamber intraocular lens		progressive care unit protective care unit
PCKD	polycystic kidney disease	PCV	packed cell volume
PCL	pacing cycle length	PCWP	pulmonary capillary wedge pressure
	posterior chamber lens	PCX	paracervical
	posterior cruciate ligament	PCXR	portable chest radiograph
	proximal collateral ligament	PCZ	procarbazine prochlorperazine
PCM	protein-calorie malnutrition	PD	interpupillary distance panic disorder
PCMX	chloroxylenol		Parkinson's disease
PCN	penicillin		percutaneous drain
	percutaneous nephrostomy		peritoneal dialysis
PCNL	percutaneous nephrostolithotomy		personality disorder poorly differentiated
PCNT	percutaneous nephrostomy tube		postural drainage prism diopter
PCO	polycystic ovary		progressive disease
PCO₂	partial pressure (tension) of carbon dioxide, artery	P/D PDA	pupillary distance packs per day (cigarettes) parenteral drug abuser patent ductus arteriosus

	posterior descending (coronary) artery		pedal edema
			physical examination
PDC	private diagnostic clinic		physical exercise
PD&C	postural drainage and clapping		plasma exchange
			pleural effusion
PDCA	Plan-Do-Check-Act (process improvement)		polyethylene
			pressure equalization
PDD	cisplatin		pulmonary edema
PDE	paroxysmal dyspnea on exertion		pulmonary embolism
		P_1E_1®	epinephrine 1%, pilocarpine 1% ophthalmic solution
	pulsed Doppler echocardiography		
PDFC	premature dead female child	P&E	prep and enema
		PEA	pelvic examination under anesthesia
PDGF	platelet derived growth factor	PEARL	pupils equal accommodation, reactive to light
PDGXT	predischarge graded exercise test		
PDL	poorly differentiated lymphocytic		pupils equal and reactive to light
	postures of daily living	PEARLA	pupils equal and react to light and accommodation
	progressively diffused leukoencephalopathy		
PDL-D	poorly differentiated lymphocytic-diffuse	PEB	cisplatin, etoposide, and bleomycin
PDL-N	poorly differentiated lymphocytic-nodular	PECCE	planned extracapsular cataract extraction
PDMC	premature dead male child	PECHR	peripheral exudative choroidal hemorrhagic retinopathy
PDN	prednisone		
	private duty nurse	PECHO	prostatic echogram
PD & P	postural drainage and percussion	PECO₂	mixed expired carbon dioxide tension
PDR	*Physician's Desk Reference*	PEDD	proton-electron dipole-dipole
	postdelivery room	PEDI DEG	pediatric deglycerolized red blood cells
	proliferative diabetic retinopathy	PEDO	pedodontist
		Peds.	pediatrics
PDRcVH	proliferative diabetic retinopathy with vitreous hemorrhage	PEEP	positive end-expiratory pressure
		PEF	peak expiratory flow
PDS	pain dysfunction syndrome	PEFR	peak expiratory flow rate
	polydioxanone suture	PEG	percutaneous endoscopic gastrostomy
PDT	photodynamic therapy		pneumoencephalogram
PDU	pulsed Doppler ultrasonography		polyethylene glycol
		PEG-ELS	polyethylene glycol and iso-osmolar electrolyte solution
PDW	platelet distribution width		
PE	cisplatin and etoposide		

PEGG	Parent Education and Guidance Group	PET	poor exercise tolerance
PEJ	percutaneous endoscopic jejunostomy		positron-emission tomography
			pre-eclamptic toxemia
PEK	punctate epithelial keratopathy		pressure equalizing tubes
		PETN	pentaerythritol tetranitrate
PEM	protein-energy malnutrition	PEx	physical examination
		PF	patellofemoral
PEMA	phenylethylmalonamide		peripheral fields
PEMS	physical, emotional, mental, and safety		plantar flexion
			power factor
PEN	parenteral and enteral nutrition		preservative free
			prostatic fluid
PENS	percutaneous epidural nerve stimulator	PF3	platelet factor 3
		PF4	repligen
PEO	progressive external ophthalmoplegia	16PF	The Sixteen Personality Factors test
PEP	pre-ejection period	PFA	foscarnet (phosphonoformatic acid)
	protein electrophoresis		
PER	pediatric emergency room	PFB	potential for breakdown
		PFC	permanent flexure contracture
	protein efficiency ratio		
PERC	perceptual		persistent fetal circulation
	percutaneous	P FEEDS	after feedings
perf.	perfect	PFFD	proximal femoral focal deficiency (defect)
	perforation		
Peri Care	perineum care	PFFFP	Pall filtered fresh frozen plasma
PERIO	periodontitis		
peri-pads	perineal pads	PFGE	pulsed field gel electrophoresis
PERL	pupils equal, reactive to light	PFJS	patellofemoral joint syndrome
per os	by mouth (this is a dangerous abbreviation as it is read as left eye)	PFM	primary fibromyalgia
			porcelain fused to metal
PERR	pattern evoked retinal response	PFO	patent foramen ovule
		PFPC	Pall filtered packed cells
PERRL	pupils equal, round, and reactive to light	PFR	parotid flow rate
			peak flow rate
PERRLA	pupils equal, round, reactive to light and accommodation	PFRC	plasma-free red cells
		PFROM	pain-free range of motion
		PFS	prefilled syringe
PERRRLA	pupils equal, round, regular, react to light and accommodation		pulmonary function studies (study)
		PFT	pulmonary function test
PES	pre-excitation syndrome	PFU	plaque-forming unit
	pseudoexfoliation syndrome	PFW	pHisoHex® face wash
		PFWB	Pall filtered whole blood
peSPL	peak equivalent sound pressure level	PG	paged in hospital
			paregoric

	paregoric		left eye
	phosphatidylglycerol	PHAL	peripheral hyperalimenta-
	picogram (pg)		tion
	polygalacturonate	PHAR	pharmacist
	pregnant		pharmacy
PGA	prostaglandin A		pharynx
PGE	posterior gastroen-	Pharm	Pharmacy
	terostomy	PharmD	Doctor of Pharmacy
PGE$_1$	alprostadil (prostaglandin	PHC	primary hepatocellular
	E$_1$)		carcinoma
PGE$_2$	dinoprostone	PHD	Public Health Department
	(prostaglandin E$_2$)	PhD	Doctor of Philosophy
PGF	paternal grandfather	PHH	posthemorrhagic
PGF$_{2\alpha}$	dinoprost (prostaglandin		hydrocephalus
	F$_{2\alpha}$)	PHI	phosphohexose isomerase
PGGF	paternal great-grandfather		prehospital index
PGGM	paternal great-	PHIS	posthead injury syndrome
	grandmother	PHL	Philadelphia
PGH	pituitary growth hormones		(chromosome)
PGI	potassium, glucose, and	PHN	postherpetic neuralgia
	insulin		public health nurse
PGI$_2$	epoprostenol		Puritan® heated nebulizer
PGL	persistent generalized	PHNI	pinhole no improvement
	lymphadenopathy	PHP	pseudohypoparathy-
PGM	paternal grandmother		roidism
PGP	paternal grandparent	PHPT	primary hyperparathy-
PgR	progesterone receptor		roidism
PGU	postgonococcal urethritis	PHPV	persistent hyperplastic
PGY-1	post-graduate year one		primary vitreous
pH	hydrogen ion	PHR	peak heart rate
	concentration	PHS	partial hospitalization
PH	past history		program
	personal history		US Public Health Service
	pinhole	PHT	phenytoin
	poor health		portal hypertension
	pubic hair		primary hyperthyroidism
	public health		pulmonary hypertension
Ph^1	Philadelphia chromosome	PHx	past history
PHA	arterial pH	Phx	pharynx
	passive hemagglutinating	PI	package insert
	peripheral hyperalimenta-		pancreatic insufficiency
	tion		Pearl Index
	phytohemagglutinin		peripheral iridectomy
	antigen		poison ivy
	postoperative holding area		postinjury
PHACO	phacoemulsification		premature infant
PHACO	phacoemulsification of the		present illness
OD	right eye		pulmonary infarction
PHACO OS	phacoemulsification of the	P & I	probe and irrigation

PIAT	Peabody Individual Achievement Test	PIPB	performance index phonetic balance
PIC	peripherally inserted catheter	PIPIDA	N-para-isopropyl-acetanilide-iminodiacetic acid
PICA	Porch Index of Communicative Ability	PIQ	Performance Intelligence Quotient (part of Wechsler tests)
	posterior inferior cerebellar artery		
	posterior inferior communicating artery	PISA	phase invariant signature algorithm
PICC	peripherally inserted central catheter	PIT	patellar inhibition test
			Pitocin®
PICU	pediatric intensive care unit		Pitressin® (this is a dangerous abbreviation)
PID	pelvic inflammatory disease		pituitary
		PITP	pseudo-idiopathic thrombocytopenic purpura
	prolapsed intervertebral disc		
	proportional-integral-derivative (controller)	PITR	plasma iron turnover rate
		PIV	peripheral intravenous
PIE	pulmonary infiltration with eosinophilia	PIVD	protruded intervertebral disc
	pulmonary interstitial emphysema	PIVKA	proteins induced by vitamin K absence
PIF	peak inspiratory flow	PIWT	partially impacted wisdom teeth
PIFG	poor intrauterine fetal growth		
		PJB	premature junctional beat
PIG	pertussis immune globulin	PJC	premature junctional contractions
PIGI	pregnancy-induced glucose intolerance	PJS	peritoneojugular shunt
			Peutz-Jeghers syndrome
PIH	preventricular intraventricular hemorrhage	PK	penetrating keratoplasty
		PKB	prone knee bend
	pregnancy induced hypertension	PKD	polycystic kidney disease
		PKP	penetrating keratoplasty
PIMS	programmable implantable medication system	PK Test	Prausnitz-Küstner transfer test
PIO	pemoline	PKU	phenylketonuria
PIO₂	partial pressure of inspired O_2	pk yrs	pack-years (smoking one pack of cigarettes a day for one year is termed 1 pack-year of smoking, thus 2 packs a day for 20 years would be 40 pack-years)
PIOK	poikilocytosis		
PI-PB	performance intensity-phonemically balanced		
PIP	peak inspiratory pressure		
	postinfusion phlebitis	PL	light perception
	proximal interphalangeal (joint)		palmaris longus
			place

	placebo		evening
	plantar		pacemaker
	transpulmonary pressure		particulate matter
PLA	Plasma-Lyte A®		petit mal
	product license application		physical medicine
			polymyositis
PLAP	placental alkaline phosphatase		poor metabolizers
			post mortem
PLAX	parasternal long axis		presents mainly
PLBO	placebo		pretibial myxedema
PLC	pityriasis lichenoides chronica		primary motivation
			prostatic massage
PLED	periodic lateralizing epileptiform discharge	PMA	premenstrual asthma
			Prinzmetal's angina
PLEVA	pityriasis lichenoides et varioliformis acuta	PMB	polymorphonuclear basophil (leukocytes)
			polymyxin B
PLFC	premature living female child		postmenopausal bleeding
		PMC	premature mitral closure
PLH	paroxysmal localized hyperhidrosis		pseudomembranous colitis
		PMCP	para-monochlorophenol
PLIF	posterior lumbar interbody fusion		perinatal mortality counseling program
PLL	prolymphocytic leukemia	PMCT	perinatal mortality counseling team
PLM	Plasma-Lyte M®		
PLMC	premature living male child	PMD	perceptual motor development
PLMS	periodic limb movements during sleep		primary myocardial disease
			primidone
PLN	pelvic lymph node		private medical doctor
	popliteal lymph node	PM/DM	polymyositis and dermatomyositis
PLOSA	physiologic low stress angioplasty		
		PME	polymorphonuclear esosinophil (leukocytes)
PLP	partial laryngopharyngectomy		
			postmenopausal estrogen
PLPH	post-lumbar puncture headache	PMEALS	after meals
		PMEC	pseudomembranous enterocolitis
PLR	pupillary light reflex		
PLS	plastic surgery	PMF	progressive massive fibrosis
	Preschool Language Scale		
	primary lateral sclerosis		pupils mid-position, fixed
PLSO	posterior leafspring orthosis	PMH	past medical history
PLSURG	plastic surgery	PMI	past medical illness
PLT	platelet		patient medication instructions
PLT EST	platelet estimate		
plts	platelets		plea of mental incompetence
PLV	posterior left ventricular		
PLX	plexus		point of maximal impulse
PM	afternoon		

	posterior myocardial infarction		postnasal
			postnatal
PML	polymorphonuclear leukocytes		practical nurse
			premie nipple
	premature labor		primary nurse
	progressive multifocal leukoencephalopathy		progress note
			pyelonephritis
PMMA	polymethylmethacrylate	P & N	psychiatry and neurology
PMMF	pectoralis major myocutaneous flat	PNAB	percutaneous needle aspiration biopsy
PMN	polymodal nociceptors	PNAS	prudent no salt added
	polymorphonuclear leukocyte	PNB	percutaneous needle biopsy
PMNN	polymorphonuclear neutrophil		premature newborn
			premature nodal beat
PMO	postmenopausal osteoporosis		prostate needle biopsy
pmol	picomole	PNC	penicillin
PMP	pain management program		peripheral nerve conduction
	previous menstrual period		premature nodal contraction
	psychotropic medication plan		prenatal care
			prenatal course
PMPO	postmenopausal palpable ovary		Psychiatric Nurse Clinician
PMR	pacemaker rhythm	PND	paroxysmal nocturnal dyspnea
	polymorphic reticulosis		pelvic node dissection
	polymyalgia rheumatica		postnasal drip
PM&R	physical medicine and rehabilitation		pregnancy, not delivered
PMS	periodic movements of sleep	PNE	peripheral neuroepithe-lioma
	post-marketing surveillance	PNET	primitive neuroectodermal tumors
	postmenopausal syndrome	PNET-MB	primitive neuroectodermal tumors-medullo-blastoma
	premenstrual syndrome		
PMT	premenstrual tension		
PMTS	premenstrual tension syndrome	PNF	proprioceptive neuromuscular fasciculation reaction
PMV	prolapse of mitral valve		
PMW	pacemaker wires	PNH	paroxysmal nocturnal hemoglobinuria
PN	parenteral nutrition	PNI	peripheral nerve injury
	percussion note		prognostic nutrition index
	percutaneous nephrosonogram	PNL	percutaneous nephrostolithotomy
	periarteritis nodosa	PNMG	persistent neonatal myasthenia gravis
	pneumonia		
	polyarteritis nodosa	PNP	peak negative pressure
	poorly nourished		

	Pediatric Nurse Practitioner		(M-protein), and skin changes
	progressive nuclear palsy	POF	position of function
	purine nucleoside	P of I	proof of illness
	phosphorylase	POG	Pediatric Oncology Group
PNS	partial nonprogressing stroke		Penthrane®-oxygen gas (nitrous oxide)
	peripheral nerve stimulator		products of gestation
	peripheral nervous system	POH	personal oral hygiene
	practical nursing student	POHA	preoperative holding area
PNT	percutaneous nephrostomy tube	POHI	physically or otherwise health impaired
pnthx	pneumothorax	POHS	presumed ocular
PNU	protein nitrogen units		histoplasmosis
PNV	postoperative nausea and vomiting		syndrome
		POI	Personal Orientation Inventory
	prenatal vitamins		postoperative instructions
Pnx	pneumonectomy	POIK	poikilocytosis
	pneumothorax	POL	premature onset of labor
PO	by mouth (*per os*)	POLY	polychromic erythrocytes
	phone order		polymorphonuclear
	postoperative		leukocyte
P_{O_2}	partial pressure (tension) of oxygen, artery	POLY-CHR	polychromatophilia
PO_4	phosphate	POM	pain on motion
POA	pancreatic oncofetal antigen		polyoximethylene
POACH	prednisone, vincristine, doxorubicin,		prescription-only medication
	cyclophosphamide, and	POMC	pro-opiomelanocortin
	cytarabine	POMP	prednisone, vincristine, methotrexate, and
POAG	primary open-angle glaucoma		mercaptopurine
POB	phenoxybenzamine	POMR	problem-oriented medical record
	place of birth	POMS	Profile of Mood States
POC	plans of care	PONI	postoperative narcotic infusion
	position of comfort		
	postoperative care	PONV	postoperative nausea and vomiting
	product of conception		
POD	pacing on demand	POOH	postoperative open heart (surgery)
	polycystic ovarian disease		
POD 1	postoperative day one	POP	pain on palpation
POE	position of ease		persistent occipitoposte-
POEMS	plasma cell dyscrasia with		rior
	polyneuropathy,		plaster of paris
	organomegaly,		popiliteal
	endocrinopathy,	POp	postoperative
	monoclonal protein	poplit	popliteal

POR	problem-oriented record		phenylpropanolamine
PORP	partial ossicular replacement prosthesis		phenylpyruvic acid
			postpartum amenorrhea
PORT	perioperative respiratory therapy	PP&A	palpation, percussion, and auscultation
	portable	PPAS	post-polio atrophy syndrome
	postoperative respiratory therapy	PPB	parts per billion
POS	parosteal osteosarcoma		positive pressure breathing
	physician's order sheet		
	positive	PPBE	postpartum breast engorgment
poss	possible		
post	post mortem examination (autopsy)	PPBS	post prandial blood sugar
		PPC	progressive patient care
post op	postoperative	PPD	packs per day
Post Sag D	posterior sagittal diameter		posterior polymorphous dystrophy
			postpartum day
post tib	posterial tibial		purified protein derivative (of tuberculin)
POT	peak occupancy time		
	plans of treatment	P & PD	percussion & postural drainage
	potential		
POU	placenta, ovaries, and uterus	PPD-B	purified protein derivative, Battey
POW	prisoner of war	PPD-S	purified protein derivative, standard
POX	pulse oximeter (reading)		
PP	near point of accommodation	PPF	plasma protein fraction
	paradoxical pulse	PPG	photoplethysmography
	partial upper and lower dentures		postprandial glucose
	pedal pulse	PPGI	psychophysiologic gastrointestinal (reaction)
	peripheral pulses		
	pin prick	PPH	postpartum hemorrhage
	plasmapheresis		primary pulmonary hypertension
	plaster of paris		
	poor person	PPHN	persistent pulmonary hypertension of the newborn
	posterior pituitary		
	postpartum	PPI	benzylpenicilloylpolysine
	postprandial		patient package insert
	presenting part		Present Pain Intensity
	private patient	PPK	population pharmaco-kinetics
	protoporphyria		
	proximal phalanx	PPL	pars plana lensectomy
	pulse pressure	PPLO	pleuro-pneumonia-like organisms
	push pills		
P&P	pins and plaster	PPM	parts per million
	policy and procedure		permanent pacemaker
PPA	palpation, percussion, and auscultation	PPMA	post-poliomyelitis muscular atrophy

PPMS	psychophysiologic musculoskeletal (reaction)		partial remission
			patient relations
			per rectum
PPN	peripheral parenteral nutrition		premature
			profile
PPNAD	primary pigmented nodular adrenocortical disease		progressive resistance
			prolonged remission
			Protestant
PPNG	penicillinase producing *Neisseria gonorrhoeae*		Puerto Rican
			pulmonic regurgitation
PPO	prefered provider organization		pulse rate
		P=R	pupils equal in size and reaction
PPOB	postpartum obstetrics		
PPP	pedal pulse present	P & R	pelvic and rectal
	peripheral pulses palpable (present)		pulse and respiration
		PR-2	Bennett pressure ventilator
	postpartum psychosis		
	protamine paracoagulation phenomenon	PRA	plasma renin activity
		PRAT	platelet radioactive antiglobulin test
PPPBL	peripheral pulses palpable both legs		
		PRBC	packed red blood cells
PPPG	postprandial plasma glucose	PRC	packed red cells
			peer review committee
PPR	patient progress record	PRCA	pure red cell aplasia
PPRC	Physician Payment Review Commission	PRD	polycystic renal disease
		PRE	passive resistance exercises
PPROM	prolonged premature rupture of membranes		progressive resistive exercise
PPS	peripheral pulmonary stenosis		proton relaxation enhancement
	postpartum sterilization	Pred	prednisone
	prospective payment system	preg	Pregestimil®
		PREMIE	premature infant
PPSS	peripheral protein sparing solution	pre-op	before surgery
PPT	person, place, and time	prep	prepare for surgery
PPTL	postpartum tubal ligation		preposition
PPU	perforated peptic ulcer	PRERLA	pupils round, equal, react to light and accommodation
PPV	pars plana vitrectomy		
	positive predictive value		
PPVT	Peabody Picture Vocabulary Test	prev	prevent
			previous
PQ	pronator quadratus	PRFN	percutaneous radio frequency
PQOCN	Psychiatric Questionnaire Obsessive-Compulsive Neurosis		
		PRG	phleborheogram
		PRH	past relevant history
PR	far point of accommodation		preretinal hemorrhage
		PRI	Pain Rating Index
	pack removal		Patient Review Instrument

prim	primary		prosthesis
PRIMIP	primipara (1st pregnancy)	PROT	protrusive relationship
PR interval	part of the electrocardiographic cycle from onset of atrial depolarization on onset of ventricular depolarization	REL	
		prov	provisional
		PROVIMI	proteins, vitamins, and minerals
		PROX	proximal
PRISM	Pediatric Risk of Mortality Score	PRP	panretinal photocoagulation
PRK	photorefractive keratectomy		patient recovery plan
			penicllinase-resistant penicillin
PRL	prolactin		pityriasis rubra pilaris
PRLA	pupils react to light and accommodation		polyribose ribitol phosphate
PRM	partial rebreathing mask		progressive rubella panencephalitis
	phosphoribomutase		
	photoreceptor membrane	PrP	prion protein
	prematurely ruptured membrane	PRP-D	*Haemophilus influenzae,* type b diphtheria conjugate vaccine
	primidone		
PRM-SDX	pyrimethamine sulfadoxine	PRPP	5-phosphoribosyl-1-pyrophosphate
PRN	as occasion requires	PRRE	pupils round regular, and equal
PRO	Professional Review Organization		
		PRRERLA	pupils round, regular, equal; react to light and accommodation
	pronation		
	protein		
	prothrombin	PRSs	positive rolandic spikes
prob	probable	PRT	protamine response test
PROCTO	procotoscopic	PRTH-C	prothrombin time control
	proctology	PRV	polycythemia rubra vera
PROG	prognathism	PRVEP	pattern reversal visual evoked potentials
	prognosis		
	program	PRW	polymerized ragweed
	progressive	PRX	panoramic facial x-ray
PROM	passive range of motion	PRZ	prazepam
	premature rupture of membranes	PRZF	pyrazofurin
		PS	paradoxic sleep
ProMACE	prednisone, methotrexate, calcium leucovorin, doxorubicin, cyclophosphamide, and etoposide		paranoid schizophrenia
			pathologic stage
			performance status
			peripheral smear
			physical status
Promy	promyelocyte		plastic surgery (surgeon)
PRO MYELO	promyelocytes		pressure support
			protective services
PRON	pronation		pulmonary stenosis
PROS	prostate		pyloric stenosis

	serum from pregnant women	PSF	posterior spinal fusion
			encephalopathy
P/S	polyunsaturated to saturated fatty acids ratio	PSG	polysomnogram
		PSIG	pounds per square inch gauge
P & S	pain and suffering	PSGN	post-streptococcal glomerulonephritis
	paracentesis and suction		
PS I	healthy patient with localized pathological process	PSH	past surgical history
			post spinal headache
		PSI	Physiologic Stability Index
PS II	a patient with mild to moderate systemic disease		pounds per square inch
		PSIS	posterior superior iliac spine
PS III	a patient with severe systemic disease limiting activity but not incapacitating		
		PSM	presystolic murmur
		PSMF	protein-sparing modified fasting (Blackburn diet)
PS IV	a patient with incapacitating systemic disease	P/sore	pressure sore
		PSP	pancreatic spasmolytic peptide
PS V	moribund patient not expected to live (These are American Society of Anesthesiologists' physical status patient classifications. Emergency operations are designated by "E" after the classification.)		phenolsulfonphthalein
			photostimulable phosphor
			progressive supranuclear palsy
		PSRBOW	premature spontaneous rupture of bag of waters
		PSS	painful shoulder syndrome
			physiologic saline solution (0.9% sodium chloride)
PSA	product selection allowed		
	prostate-specific antigen		progressive systemic sclerosis
PsA	psoriatic arthritis		
PSC	Pediatric Symptom Checklist	PST	paroxysmal supraventricular tachycardia
	posterior subcapsular cataract		platelet survival time
	primary sclerosing cholangitis	PSV	pressure supported ventilation
PSCC	posterior subcapsular cataract	PSVT	paroxysmal supraventricular tachycardia
PSCH	peripheral stem cell harvest	PSW	psychiatric social worker
		PSY	pre-sexual youth
PSCP	posterior subcapsular precipitates	PT	cisplatin
			parathormone
PSCT	peripheral stem cell transplant		parathyroid
			paroxysmal tachycardia
PSCU	pediatric special care unit		patient
PSE	portal systemic		phenytoin

	phototoxicity		coronary rotational atherectomy
	physical therapy		
	pine tar	PTD	period to discharge
	pint		permanent and total disability
	posterior tibial		persistent trophoblastic disease
	preterm		
	prothrombin time		pharmacy to dose
P&T	paracentesis and tubing (of ears)		prior to delivery
	peak and trough	PTDP	permanent transvenous demand pacemaker
	permanent and total		
PTA	percutaneous transluminal angioplasty	PTE	pretibial edema
	Physical Therapy Assistant		proximal tibial epiphysis
			pulmonary thromboembolism
	plasma thromboplastin antecedent	PTED	pulmonary thromboembolic disease
	post-traumatic amnesia	PTFE	polytetrafluoroethylene
	pretreatment anxiety	PTG	parathyroid gland
	prior to admission		teniposide
	pure-tone average	PTH	parathyroid hormone
PTB	patellar tendon bearing		post-transfusion hepatitis
	prior to birth		prior to hospitalization
	pulmonary tuberculosis	PTHC	percutaneous transhepatic cholangiography
PTBA	percutaneous transluminal balloon angioplasty	PTJV	percutaneous transtracheal jet ventilation
PTBD-EF	percutaneous transhepatic biliary drainage—enteric feeding	PTK	phototherapeutic keratectomy
PTBS	post-traumatic brain syndrome	PTL	pre-term labor
			Sodium Pentothal®
PTB-SC-SP	patellar tendon bearing-supracondylar-suprapatellar	PTLD	post-transplant lymphoproliferative disorder
PTC	patient to call	PTMDF	pupils, tension, media, disc, and fundus
	percutaneous transhepatic cholangiography	PTNB	preterm newborn
	plasma thromboplastin components	PTNM	postsurgical resection-pathologic staging of cancer
	prior to conception		
	pseudotumor cerebri	PTO	please turn over
PT-C	prothrombin time control	PTP	posterior tibial pulse
PTCA	percutaneous transluminal coronary angioplasty	PTPM	post-traumatic progressive myelopathy
PTCL	peripheral T-cell lymphoma	PTPN	peripheral (vein) total parenteral nutrition
PTCR	percutaneous transluminal coronary recanalization	PTR	paratesticular rhabdomyosarcoma
PTCRA	percutaneous transluminal		patella tendon reflex

	patient to return	PUO	pyrexia of unknown origin
	prothrombin time ratio		
PT-R	prothrombin time ratio	PUP	percutaneous ultrasonic pyelolithotomy
PTRA	percutaneous transluminal renal angioplasty	PU/PL	partial upper and lower dentures
PTS	patellar tendon suspension		
	Pediatric Trauma Score	PUPP	pruritic urticarial papules and plaque of pregnancy
	permanent threshold shift		
	prior to surgery		
PTSD	post-traumatic stress disorder	PUS	percutaneous ureteral stent
PTT	partial thromboplastin time	PUVA	psoralen-ultraviolet-light (treatment)
	platelet transfusion therapy	PV	papillomavirus
PTT-C	partial thromboplastin time control		per vagina
			plasma volume
PTU	pain treatment unit		polio vaccine
	propylthiouracil		polycythemia vera
PTV	posterior tibial vein		popliteal vein
PTWTKG	patient's weight in kilograms		portal vein
			postvoiding
PTX	parathyroidectomy		pulmonary vein
	pelvic traction	P&V	peak and valley (this is a dangerous abbreviation) use peak and trough
	pneumothorax		
PTZ	pentylenetetrazol		
	phenothiazine		pyloroplasty and vagotomy
PU	pelvic-ureteric		
	pelviureteral	PVA	polyvinyl alcohol
	peptic ulcer		Prinzmetal's variant angina
	pregnancy urine		
PUA	pelvic (examination) under anesthesia	PVAD	prolonged venous access devices
PUBS	percutaneous umbilical blood sampling	PVB	cisplatin, vinblastine, and bleomycin
PUC	pediatric urine collector		premature ventricular beat
PUD	peptic ulcer disease	PVC	polyethylene vacuum cup
	percutaneous ureteral dilatation		polyvinyl chloride
			postvoiding cystogram
PUE	pyrexia of unknown etiology		premature ventricular contraction
PUF	pure ultrafiltration		pulmonary venous congestion
PUFA	polyunsaturated fatty acids	$Pvco_2$	partial pressure (tension) of carbon dioxide, vein
pul.	pulmonary		
PULSE OX	pulse oximetry	PVD	patient very disturbed
			peripheral vascular disease
PUN	plasma urea nitrogen		
PUNL	percutaneous ultrasonic nephrolithotripsy		posterior vitreous detachment

	premature ventricular depolarization	PVS	pulse-volume recording percussion, vibration and suction peripheral vascular surgery peritoneovenous shunt persistent vegetative state
PVE	perivenous encephalomy-elitis premature ventricular extrasystole prosthetic value endocarditis		
PVF	peripheral visual field		Plummer-Vinson
PVFS	postviral fatigue syndrome		syndrome pulmonic valve stenosis
PVH	periventricular hemorrhage	PVT	paroxysmal ventricular tachycardia
	periventricular hyperintensity		private
	pulmonary vascular	PVTT	tumor thrombus in the portal vein
	hypertension	PW	pacing wires
PVI	peripheral vascular insufficiency		patient waiting pulse width
PVK	penicillin V potassium		puncture wound
PVL	periventricular	P&W	pressures and waves
	leukomalacia	PWA	persons with AIDS
PVM	paravertebral muscle	P wave	part of the electrocardio-
	proteins, vitamins, and minerals		graphic cycle representing atrial depolarization
PVN	peripheral venous nutrition	PWB	partial weight bearing psychological well-being
PVNS	pigmented villonodular	PWI	pediatric walk-in clinic
	synovitis		posterior wall infarct
PVO	peripheral vascular occlusion	PWLV	posterior wall of left ventricle
	pulmonary venous occlusion	PWM	pokeweed mitogens
PVo₂	partial pressure (tension)	PWP	pulmonary wedge pressure
	of oxygen, vein	PWS	port-wine stain
PVOD	pulmonary vascular	PWV	polistes wasp venom
	obstructive disease	Px	physical exam
PVP	cisplatin and etoposide		pneumothorax
	peripheral venous		prognosis
	pressure	PXE	pseudoxanthoma
	polyvinylpyrrolidone		elasticum
P-VP-B	cisplatin, etoposide, and	PXF	pseudoexfoliation
	bleomycin	PXS	dental prophylaxis
PVR	peripheral vascular		(cleaning)
	resistance	PY	pack years (see pk yrs)
	postvoiding residual	PYE	person-years of exposure
	proliferative	PYHx	packs per year history
	vitreoretinopathy	PYP	pyrophosphate
	pulmonary vascular	PYP®	technetium Tc 99m
	resistance		pyrophosphate kit

PZ	peripheral zone	
PZA	pyrazinamide	
PZI	protamine zinc insulin	

Q

q	every
QA	quality assurance
QAC	before every meal
QALYs	quality adjusted life years
QAM	every morning (this is a dangerous abbreviation)
QC	quad cane
	quality control
	quick catheter
QCA	quantitative coronary angiography
QCT	quantitative computed tomography
qd	every day (this is a dangerous abbreviation as it is read as four times daily)
QE	quinidine effect
q4h	every four hours
qh	every hour
qhs	every night (this is a dangerous abbreviation as it is read as every hour)
qid	four times daily
QIDM	four times daily with meals and at bedtime
QIG	quantitative immunoglobulins
QL	quality of life
QLI	Quality of Life Index
QMI	Q wave myocardial infarction
QMRP	qualified mental retardation professional
QMT	quantitative muscle testing

q.n.	every night (this is a dangerous abbreviation as it is read as every hour)
q.n.s.	quantity not sufficient
qod	every other day (this is a dangerous abbreviation as it is read as every day or four times a day)
qoh	every other hour (this is a dangerous abbreviation as it is read as every day or four times a day)
qohs	every other night (this is a dangerous abbreviation as it is not recognized)
QOL	quality of life
QON	every other night (this is a dangerous abbreviation)
qpm	every evening (this is a dangerous abbreviation)
QP/QS	ratio of pulmonary blood to systemic blood flow
QR	quiet room
QRS	part of electrocardiographic wave representing ventricular depolarization
Q.S.	every shift
	sufficient quantity
Qs/Qt	intrapulmonary shunt fraction
QSP	physiological shunt fraction
qt	quart
QTB	quadriceps tendon bearing
QTC	quantitative tip cultures
QUAD	quadrant
	quadriceps
	quadriplegic
QU	quiet
QUART	quadrantectomy, axillary dissection, and radiotherapy
QWB	Quality of Well-Being (scale)

qwk	once a week (this is a dangerous abbreviation)		skeletal hyperostosis
		RAE	right atrial enlargement
		RAEB	refractory anemia, erythroblastic
		RAF	rapid atrial fibrillation
		RAFT	Rehabilitative Addicted Family Treatment

R

		RAG	room air gas
R	rate	RAH	right atrial hypertrophy
	reacting	RAIU	radioactive iodine uptake
	rectal	RALT	routine admission laboratory tests
	rectum		
	regular	RAM	radioactive material
	regular insulin		rapid alternating movements
	resistant		rectus abdominis myocutaneous
	respiration		
	right	RAN	resident's admission notes
	roentgen	R₂AN	second year resident's admission notes
	rub		
Ⓡ	registered trademark	RAO	right anterior oblique
	right	RAP	right atrial pressure
RA	rales	RAPA	radial artery pseudoaneurysm
	repeat action		
	retinoic acid	RAQ	right anterior quadrant
	rheumatoid arthritis	RAPD	relative afferent pupillary defect
	right arm		
	right atrium	RAS	recurrent aphthous stomatitis
	right auricle		renal artery stenosis
	room air		reticular activating system
RAA	renin-angiotensin-aldoste-rone	RASE	rapid-acquisition spin echo
RAAS	renin-angiotensin-aldoste-rone system	RAST	radioallergosorbent test
		RAT	right anterior thigh
RABG	room air blood gas	RA test	test for rheumatoid factor
RAC	right atrial catheter	RATx	radiation therapy
RACCO	right anterior caudocranial oblique	R(AW)	airway resistance
		RB	retinoblastoma
RACT	recalcified whole-blood activated clotting time		retrobulbar
			right buttock
RAD	ionizing radiation unit	R & B	right and below
	radical	RBA	right basilar artery
	radiology		right brachial artery
	reactive airway disease	RBB	right breast biopsy
	right axis deviation	RBBB	right bundle branch block
RADISH	rheumatoid arthritis diffuse idiopathic	RBBX	right breast biopsy examination
		RBC	red blood cell (count)

RBCD	right border cardiac dullness	RCS	repeat cesarean section
			reticulum cell sarcoma
RBCM	red blood cell mass	RCT	randomized clinical trial
RBC s/f	red blood cells spun filtration		Registered Care Technologist
RBCV	red blood cell volume		root canal therapy
RBD	right border of dullness		Rorschach Content Test
RBE	relative biologic effectiveness	RCV	red cell volume
		RD	Raynaud's disease
RBF	renal blood flow		reflex decay
RBG	random blood glucose		Registered Dietitian
RBL	Roche Biomedical Laboratory		renal disease
			respiratory disease
RBOW	rupture bag of water		retinal detachment
RBP	retinol-binding protein		Reye's disease
RBS	random blood sugar		right deltoid
RBT	rational behavior therapy		ruptured disc
RBV	right brachial vein	RDA	recommended daily allowance
RC	race		
	Red Cross	RDCS	Registered Diagnostic Cardiac Sonographer
	report called		
	right coronary	RDEA	right deviation of electrical axis
	Roman Catholic		
	rotator cuff	RDG	right dorsogluteal
R/C	reclining chair	RDH	Registered Dental Hygienist
RCA	radionuclide cerebral angiogram		
		RDI	respiratory disturbance index
	right coronary artery		
RCBF	regional cerebral blood flow	RDIH	right direct inguinal hernia
RCC	renal cell carcinoma	RDMS	Registered Diagnostic Medical Sonographer
RCCT	randomized controlled clinical trial		
		RDOD	retinal detachment, right eye
RCD	relative cardiac dullness		
RCE	right carotid endarterectomy	RDOS	retinal detachment, left eye
RCF	Reiter complement fixation	RDP	random donor platelets
			right dorsoposterior
RCHF	right-sided congestive heart failure	RDPE	reticular degeneration of the pigment epithelium
RCM	radiographic contrast media	RDS	research diagnostic criteria
	retinal capillary microaneurysm		respiratory distress syndrome
	right costal margin	RDT	regular dialysis (hemodialysis) treatment
RCPM	raven coloured progressive matrices		
RCPT	Registered Cardiopulmonary Technician	RDTD	referral, diagnosis, treatment, and discharge

RDVT	recurrent deep vein thrombosis		repeat
RDW	red (cell) distribution width	repol	report
		REPS	repolarization
RE	concerning	REPT	repetitions
	rectal examination		Registered Evoked Potential Technologist
	reflux esophagitis	RER	renal excretion rate
	regarding	RES	resection
	regional enteritis		resident
	reticuloendothelial		reticuloendothelial system
	retinol equivalents	RESC	resuscitation
	right ear	resp.	respirations
	right eye		respiratory
	rowing ergometer	REST	restoration
R & E	rest and exercise	RET	retention
	round and equal		reticulocyte
R ↑ E	right upper extremity		retina
RE ✔	recheck		retired
READM	readmission		return
REC	rear end collision		right esotropia
	recommend	retic	reticulocyte
	record	REV	reverse
	recovery		review
	recreation		revolutions
	recur	RF	renal failure
RECT	rectum		rheumatic fever
RED SUBS	reducing substances		rheumatoid factor
			risk factor
REE	resting energy expenditure		radiofrequency
RE-ED	re-education	R&F	radiographic and fluoroscopic
R-EEG	resting electroencephalo-gram	RFA	right femoral artery
			right frontoanterior
REEGT	Registered Electroenceph-alogram Technologist	RFE	return flow enema
		RFIPC	Rating Form of IBD (inflammatory bowel disease) Patient Concerns
REF	referred		
	refused		
	renal erythropoietic factor		
ref →	refer to	RFL	right frontolateral
Reg block	regional block anesthesia	RFLP	restriction fragment length polymorphism (patterns)
regurg	regurgitation		
rehab	rehabilitation		
REL	relative	RFM	rifampin
	religion	RFP	request for payment
REM	rapid eye movement		right frontoposterior
	recent event memory	RFS	rapid frozen section
	remission	RFT	right frontotransverse
	roentgen equivalent unit		routine fever therapy
REMS	rapid eye movement sleep	RG	right (upper outer) gluteus
REP	repair		

RGM	right gluteus medius		right iliac fossa
RGO	reciprocating gait orthosis		right index finger
Rh	Rhesus factor in blood		rigid internal fixation
RH	reduced haloperidol	RIG	rabies immune globulin
	rest home	RIH	right inguinal hernia
	retinal hemorrhage	RIJ	right internal jugular
	right hand	RIMA	right internal mammary
	right hyperphoria		anastamosis
	room humidifier	RIND	reversible ischemic
RHB	raise head of bed		neurologic defect
RH/BSO	radial hysterectomy and	RIP	radioimmunoprecipitin
	bilateral salpingo-		test
	oophorectomy		rapid infusion pump
RHC	respiration has ceased		respiratory inductance
RHD	relative hepatic dullness		plethysmograph
	rheumatic heart disease	RIPA	ristocetin-induced platelet
RHF	right heart failure		agglutination
RHG	right hand grip	RIR	right inferior rectus
RHH	right homonymous	RISA	radioactive iodinated
	hemianopsia		serum albumin
RHL	right hemisphere lesions	RIST	radioimmunosorbent test
rHmEPO	recombinant human	RK	radial keratotomy
	erythropoietin		right kidney
Rho(D)	immune globulin to an	RL	right lateral
	Rh-negative woman		right leg
			right lung
RhoGAM®	Rh$_O$ (D) immune globulin		Ringer's lactate
RHS	right hand side	R➤L	right to left
RHT	right hypertropia	RLBCD	right lower border of
RHW	radiant heat warmer		cardiac dullness
RI	regular insulin	RLC	residual lung capacity
	rooming in	RLD	related living donor
RIA	radioimmunoassay		right lateral decubitus
RIAT	radioimmune antiglobulin	RLDP	right lateral decubital
	test		position
RIC	right iliac crest	RLE	right lower extremity
	right internal carotid	RLF	retrolental fibroplasia
	(artery)	RLL	right lower lid
RICE	rest, ice, compression,		right lower lobe
	and elevation	RLN	recurrent laryngeal nerve
RICM	right intercostal margin	RLQ	right lower quadrant
RICS	right intercostal space	RLR	right lateral rectus
RICU	respiratory intensive care	RLS	restless legs syndrome
	unit		Ringer's lactate solution
RID	radial immunodiffusion	RLT	right lateral thigh
	ruptured intervertebral	RLTCS	repeat low transverse
	disc		cesarean section
RIE	rocket immunoelectro-	RM	radical mastectomy
	phoresis		repetitions maximum
RIF	rifampin		

	respiratory movement	RNEF	resting (radio-) nuclide ejection fraction
	room		
R&M	routine and microscopic	RNLP	Registered Nurse, license pending
RMA	Registered Medical Assistant	RNP	Registered Nurse Practitioner
	right mentoanterior		
RMCA	right main coronary artery	RNS	replacement normal saline (0.9% sodium chloride)
	right middle cerebral artery	RNST	reactive non-stress test
RMCL	right midclavicular line	RO	relative odds
RMD	rapid movement disorder		reverse osmosis
RME	resting metabolic expenditure		routine order
		R/O	rule out
	right mediolateral episiotomy	ROA	right occiput anterior
RMEE	right middle ear exploration	ROAC	repeated oral doses of activated charcoal
RMK #1	remark number 1	ROAD	reversible obstructive airway disease
RML	right mediolateral		
	right middle lobe	ROC	receiver operating characteristic
RMLE	right mediolateral episiotomy		record of contact
RMP	right mentoposterior		resident on call
RMR	resting metabolic rate		residual organic carbon
	right medial rectus	ROI	region of interest
		ROIDS	hemorrhoids
RMS	Rehabilitation Medicine Service	ROIH	right oblique inguinal hernia
	repetitive motion syndrome	ROL	right occipitolateral
RMS®	rectal morphine sulfate (suppository)	ROM	range of motion
			right otitis media
RMSB	right middle sternal border		rupture of membranes
		Romb	Romberg
RMSE	root mean square error	ROMI	rule out myocardial infarction
RMSF	Rocky Mountain spotted fever	ROMSA	right otitis media, suppurative, acute
RMT	Registered Music Therapist	ROMSC	right otitis media, suppurative, chronic
	right mentotransverse	ROP	retinopathy of prematurity
RN	Registered Nurse		right occiput posterior
	right nostril (nare)	ROPE	regional organ physical examination
R/N	renew		
RNA	radionuclide angiography	RoRx	radiation therapy
	ribonucleic acid	ROS	review of systems
RNC	Registered Nurse, Certified		rod outer segments
		ROSC	restoration of spontaneous circulation
RNCD	Registered Nurse, Chemical Dependency	ROT	remedial occupational therapy
RND	radical neck dissection		

	right occipital transverse rotator	RPT	Registered Physical Therapist
ROUL	rouleaux	RPTA	Registered Physical
RP	radial pulse		Therapist Assistant
	radiopharmaceutical	RQ	respiratory quotient
	Raynaud's phenomenon	RR	recovery room
	retinitis pigmentosa		regular respirations
	retrograde pyelogram		relative risk
RPA	radial photon absorptiometry		respiratory rate retinal reflex
	Registered Physician's Assistant	R/R	rales-rhonchi
		R&R	rate and rhythm
	right pulmonary artery		recent and remote
RPCF	Reiter protein complement fixation		recession and resection rest and recuperation
RPD	removable partial denture		remove and replace
RPE	rating of perceived exertion	RRA	radioreceptor assay
			Registered Record
RPEP	right pre-ejection period		Administrator
	retinal pigment epithelium	RRAM	rapid rhythmic alternating
RPF	relaxed pelvic floor		movements
	renal plasma flow	RRCT,	regular rate, clear tones,
RPG	retrograde pyelogram	no(m)	no murmurs
RPGN	rapidly progressive glomerulonephritis	RRE	round, regular, and equal (pupils)
RPH	retroperitoneal hemorrhage	RREF	resting radionuclide ejection fraction
RPI	reticulocyte production index	RRNA	Resident Registered Nurse Anesthetist
R.Ph.	Registered Pharmacist	rRNA	ribosomal ribonucleic acid
RPHA	reverse passive hemagglutination	RRND	right radical neck dissection
RPICCE	round pupil intracapsular cataract extraction	RROM	resistive range of motion
		RRP	radical retropubic
RPL	retroperitoneal lymphadenectomy		prostatectomy
		RRR	regular rhythm and rate
RPLND	retroperitoneal lymph node dissection	RRRN	round, regular, and react normally
RPN	renal papillary necrosis resident's progress notes	RRRsM	regular rate and rhythm without murmur
R₂PN	second year resident's progress notes	RRT	Registered Respiratory Therapist
RPO	right posterior oblique	RRVO	repair relaxed vaginal
RPP	radical perineal prostatectomy		outlet
		RS	Raynaud's syndrome
	rate-pressure product		Reiter's syndrome
RPR	rapid plasma reagin (test for syphilis)		Reye's syndrome rhythm strip
	Reiter protein reagin		right side

	Ringer's solution	RTF	ready-to-feed
R/S	rest stress		return to flow
	rupture spontaneous	RTI	reverse transcriptase
RSA	right sacrum anterior		inhibitor
	right subclavian artery	RTL	reactive to light
RSC	right subclavian	RTM	routine medical care
RScA	right scapuloanterior	RTN	renal tubular necrosis
RScP	right scapuloposterior	RTNM	retreatment staging of
rscu-PA	recombinant,		cancer
	single-chain,	RTO	return to office
	urokinase-type	RTOG	Radiation Therapy
	plasminogen activator		Oncology Group
RSDS	reflex-sympathetic	RTP	return to pharmacy
	dystrophy syndrome	rtPA	alteplase (recombinant
RSI	repetitive strain injury		tissue-type plasminogen
R-SICU	respiratory-surgical		activator)
	intensive care unit	RT (R)	Radiologic Technologist
RSO	right salpingooophorec-		(Registered)
	tomy	RTRR	return to recovery room
	right superior oblique	RTS	raised toilet seat
RSP	rapid straight pacing		real time scan
	right sacroposterior		return to sender
RSR	regular sinus rhythm	RTT	Respiratory Therapy
	relative survival rate		Technician
	right superior rectus	RT₃U	resin triiodothyronine
RSS	Russian spring-summer		uptake
	(encephalitis)	RTUS	realtime ultrasound
RST	right sacrum transverse	RTW	return to ward
RSTs	Rodney Smith tubes		return to work
RSV	respiratory syncytial virus	RTWD	return to work
	right subclavian vein		determination
RSW	right-sided weakness	RTx	radiation therapy
RT	radiation therapy	RU	routine urinalysis
	Radiologic Technologist	RU 486	mifepristone
	recreational therapy	RUA	routine urine analysis
	rectal temperature	RUE	right upper extremity
	renal transplant	RUG	retrograde urethrogram
	repetition time	RUL	right upper lobe
	respiratory therapist	RUOQ	right upper outer quadrant
	right	rupt.	ruptured
	right thigh	RUQ	right upper quadrant
R/t	related to	RURTI	recurrent upper
RTA	renal tubular acidosis		respiratory tract
	road traffic accident		infection
RTC	return to clinic	RUSB	right upper sternal border
	round the clock	RV	rectovaginal
RTCA	ribavirin		residual volume
RTER	return to emergency room		respiratory volume
rt. ↟ ext.	right upper extremity		return visit

	right ventricle		prescription
	rubella vaccine		radiotherapy
RVA	right ventricular apex		take
RVAD	right ventricular assist device		therapy
			treatment
RVD	relative vertebral density	RXN	reaction
RVE	right ventricular enlargement	RXT	radiation therapy
			right exotropia
RVEDP	right ventricular end-diastolic pressure		
RVET	right ventricular ejection time		

S

RVF	Rift Valley fever		
	right ventricular function		
RVG	radionuclide ventriculography		
	right ventrogluteal		
RVH	renovascular hypertension	S	sacral
	right ventricular hypertrophy		second (s)
			Semilente Insulin®
RVIDd	right ventricle internal dimension diastole		sensitive
			serum
RVL	right vastus lateralis		single
RVO	relaxed vaginal outlet		sister
	retinal vein occlusion		son
	right ventricular outflow		subjective findings
	right ventricular overactivity		suction
			sulfur
RVOT	right ventricular outflow tract		supervision
		s̄	without (this is a dangerous abbreviation)
RVP	right ventricular pressure		
RVR	rapid ventricular response	S_1	first heart sound
	right ventricular rhythm	S^{-1}	hertz
RVS	rabies vaccine, adsorbed	S_2	second heart sound
RVSWI	right ventricular stroke work index	S_3	third heart sound (ventricular gallop)
RVT	renal vein thrombosis	S_4	fourth heart sound (atrial gallop)
RV/TLC	residual volume to total lung capacity ratio		
		$S_1...S_5$	sacral vertebra 1 through 5
RVV	rubella vaccine virus		
RVVT	Russell's viper venom time	SI to SIV	symbols for the first to fourth heart sounds
RW	ragweed	SA	salicylic acid
	red welt		semen analysis
R/W	return to work		sinoatrial
RWM	regional wall motion		sleep apnea
Rx	drug		Spanish American
	medication		substance abuse
	pharmacy		suicide alert

	suicide attempt	SAI	Sodium Amytal® interview
	surface area		
	surgical assistant	SAL	salicylate
	sustained action		*Salmonella*
S/A	same as	SAL 12	sequential analysis of 12 chemistry constituents
	sugar and acetone		
S&A	sugar and acetone	SAM	selective antimicrobial modulation
SAA	same as above		
SAB	serum albumin		self-administered medication
	sino-atrial block		
	spontaneous abortion		systolic anterior motion
	subarachnoid bleed	SAN	side-arm nebulizer
	subarachnoid block		sinoatrial node
SAC	serum aminoglycoside concentration		slept all night
		SANC	short arm navicular cast
	short arm cast	sang	sanguinous
	substance abuse counselor	SANS	Schedule (Scale) for the Assessment of Negative Symptoms
SACC	short arm cylinder cast		
SACH	soft ankle, cushioned heel		
	solid ankle, cushion heel	SANS	sympathetic autonomic nervous system
SACT	sinoatrial conduction time		
SAD	seasonal affective disorder	SAO	small airway obstruction
	Self-Assessment Depression (scale)	SaO₂	arterial oxygen percent saturation
	source-axis distance	SAPD	self-administration of psychotropic drugs
	subacute dialysis		
	sugar, acetone, and diacetic acid	SAPH	saphenous
		SAPS	short arm plaster splint
	sugar and acetone determination		Simplified Acute Physiology Score
	superior axis deviation	SAQ	short arc quad
SADL	simulated activities of daily living	SAR	seasonal allergic rhinitis
			Senior Assistant Resident
SADR	suspected adverse drug reaction		sexual attitudes reassessment
SADS	Schedule for Affective Disorders and Schizophrenia	SARA	sexually acquired reactive arthritis
			system for anesthetic and respiratory administration analysis
SAE	short above elbow (cast)		
SAEKG	signaled average electrocardiogram	SARAN	senior admitting resident's admission note
SAESU	Substance Abuse Evaluating Screen Unit	SARC	seasonal allergic rhinoconjunctivitis
SAF	Self-Analysis Form	SAS	saline, agent, and saline
	self-articulating femoral		scalenus anticus syndrome
Sag D	sagittal diameter		Self-rating Anxiety Scale
SAH	subarachnoid hemorrhage		short arm splint
	systemic arterial hypertension		sleep apnea syndrome

	Social Adjustment Scale	SBD	straight bag drainage
	Specific Activity Scale	SBE	short below elbow (cast)
	subarachnoid space		shortness of breath on
	sulfasalazine		exertion
SASH	saline, agent, saline, and		subacute bacterial
	heparin		endocarditis
SASP	sulfasalazine	SBFT	small bowel follow
	(salicylazosulfapyri-		through
	dine)	SBG	stand-by guard
SAT	saturated	SBGM	self blood glucose
	saturation		monitoring
	Saturday	SBI	systemic bacterial
	Senior Apperception Test		infection
	speech awareness	SBK	spinnbarkeit
	threshold	SB-LM	Stanford-Binet
	subacute thyroiditis		Intelligence Test-Form
SATL	surgical Achilles tendon		LM
	lengthening	SBO	small bowel obstruction
SATU	substance abuse treatment	SBOD	scleral buckle, right eye
	unit	SBOH	State Board of Health
SAVD	spontaneous assisted	SBOM	soybean oil meal
	vaginal delivery	SBOS	scleral buckle, left eye
SB	safety belt	SBP	school breakfast program
	sandbag		scleral buckling procedure
	seat belt		small bowel phytobezoars
	seen by		spontaneous bacterial
	Sengstaken-Blakemore		peritonitis
	(tube)		systolic blood pressure
	side bending	SBQC	small based quad cane
	sinus bradycardia	SBR	sluggish blood return
	small bowel		strict bed rest
	spina bifida	SBS	shaken baby syndrome
	stand-by		short bowel syndrome
	Stanford-Binet (test)		small bowel series
	sternal border	SBT	serum bactericidal titers
	stillbirth	SBTB	sinus breakthrough beat
	stillborn	SBTT	small bowel transit time
Sb	antimony	SBV	single binocular vision
SB+	wearing seat belt	SBX	symphysis, buttocks, and
SB−	not wearing seat belt		xiphoid
SBA	serum bactericidal activity	SC	schizophrenia
	standby angioplasty		self-care
	standby assistant		serum creatinine
	(assistance)		service connected
SBC	sensory binocular		sickle-cell
	cooperation		Snellen's chart
	single base cane		spinal cord
	standard bicarbonate		sternoclavicular
	strict bed confinement		subclavian

	subclavian catheter
	subcutaneous
	sulfur colloid
	without correction (without glasses)
SCA	sickle cell anemia
	subclavian artery
	subcutaneous abdominal (block)
SCAN	suspected child abuse and neglect
SCAT	sheep cell agglutination titer
	sickle cell anemia test
SCB	strictly confined to bed
SCBC	small cell bronchogenic carcinoma
SCBE	single-contrast barium enema
SCBF	spinal cord blood flow
SCC	sickle cell crisis
SCC	small cell carcinoma
	squamous cell carcinoma
SCCa	squamous cell carcinoma
SCCA	semi-closed circle absorber
	squamous cell carcinoma antigen
SCCI	subcutaneous continuous infusion
SCD	sequential compression device
	service connected disability
	sickle cell disease
	spinal cord disease
	subacute combined degeneration
	sudden cardiac death
ScDA	scapulodextra anterior
SCDM	soybean-casein digest medium
ScDP	scapulodextra posterior
SCE	sister chromatid exchange
SCEMIA	self-contained enzymic membrane immunoassay
SCEP	somatosensory cortical evoked potential
SCF	special care formula
SCFE	slipped capital femoral epiphysis
SCG	seismocardiography
	sodium cromoglycate
SCh	succinylcholine chloride
SCHISTO	schistocytes
SCHIZ	schizocytes
	schizophrenia
SCHLP	supracricord hemilaryngopharyngectomy
SCI	spinal cord injury
SCID	severe combined immunodeficiency disorders (disease)
	structured clinical interview for DSM-III-R
SCIPP	sacrococcygeal to inferior pubic point
SCIU	spinal cord injury unit
SCIV	subclavian intravenous
SCL	skin conductance level
	symptom checklist
SCL-90	Symptoms Checklist—90 items
ScLA	scapulolaeva anterior
SCLAX	subcostal long axis
SCLC	small-cell lung cancer
SCLE	subcutaneous lupus erythematosis
ScLP	scapulolaeva posterior
SCLs	soft contact lenses
SCM	sensation, circulation, and motion
	spondylitic caudal myelopathy
	sternocleidomastoid
SCMD	senile choroidal macular degeneration
SCN	special care nursery
SCOP	scopolamine
SCOPE	arthroscopy
SCP	sodium cellulose phosphate
	standardized care plan
SCR	special care room (seclusion room)

	spondylitic caudal radioculopathy		sodium deoxycholate
SCr	serum creatinine	SD&C	suction, dilation, and curettage
SC/RP	scaling and root planing	SDB	self-destructive behavior
SCSAX	subcostal short axis	SDC	sleep disorders center
SCT	Sertoli cell tumor	SDD	selective digestive (tract) decontamination
	sickel cell trait		
	sugar coated tablet	SDH	subdural hematoma
SCTX	static cervical traction	SDL	serum digoxin level
SCU	self-care unit		serum drug level
	special care unit		speech discrimination loss
SCUCP	small cell undifferentiated carcinoma of the prostate	S/D/M	systolic, diastolic, mean
		SD/N	signal-difference-to-noise ratio
SCUF	slow and continuous ultrafiltration	SDP	sacrodextra posterior
			single donor platelets
SCUT	schizophrenia, chronic undifferentiated type		stomach, duodenum, and pancreas
SCV	subclavian vein	SDR	selective dorsal rhizotomy
	subcutaneous vaginal (block)	SDS	same day surgery
			Self-Rating Depression Scale
SD	scleroderma		
	senile dementia		sodium dodecylsulfate
	septal defect		Speech Discrimination Score
	severely disabled		
	shoulder disarticulation	SDT	sacrodextra transversa
	single dose		speech detection threshold
	spasmodic dysphonia	SDU	step-down unit
	spontaneous delivery	SE	saline enema
	standard deviation		side effect
	standard diet		soft exudates
	sterile dressing		spin echo
	straight drainage		standard error
	streptozocin and doxorubicin		Starr-Edwards (pacemaker)
	sudden death	Se	selenium
	surgical drain	S/E	suicidal and eloper
S & D	stomach and duodenum	sec	second
S/D	systolic-diastolic ratio		secondary
SDA	sacrodextra anterior		secretary
	Seventh-Day Adventist	SECL	seclusion
	steroid-dependent asthmatic	SECPR	standard external cardiopulmonary resuscitation
SDAT	senile dementia of Alzheimer's type	SED	sedimentation
			socially and emotionally disturbed
SDB	sleep disordered breathing		spondyloepiphyseal dysplasia
SDC	serum digoxin concentration		
	Sleep Disorders Center		

sed rt	sedimentation rate		sugar free
SEER	Surveillance, Epidemiology, and End Results (program)		symptom-free
			synovial fluid
		S&F	soft and flat
SEG	segment	SF 36	Short Form 36
segs	segmented neutrophils	SFA	saturated fatty acids
SEH	spinal epidural hematomas		superficial femoral artery
	subependymal hemorrhage	SFC	spinal fluid count
		SFD	small for dates
SEI	subepithelial (comeal) infiltrate	SFEMG	single-fiber electromyography
SELFVD	sterile elective low forceps vaginal delivery	SFP	simulated fluorescence process
SEM	scanning electron microscopy		simultaneous foveal perception
	semen		spinal fluid pressure
	slow eye movement	SFPT	standard fixation preference test
	standard error of mean	SFS	split function studies
	systolic ejection murmur	SFTR	sagittal, frontal, transverse, rotation
SEMI	subendocardial myocardial infarction	SFUP	surgical follow-up
SENS	sensitivity	SFV	superficial femoral vein
	sensorium	SFW	shell fragment wound
SEP	separate	SG	salivary gland
	serum electrophoresis		scrotography
	somatosensory evoked potential		serum glucose
			skin graft
	systolic ejection period		specific gravity
SEQ	sequela		Swan-Ganz (catheter)
SER	scanning equalization radiography	SGA	small for gestational age
			substantial gainful activity (employment)
SER-IV	supination external rotation, type 4 fracture	SGC	Swan-Ganz catheter
SERO-SANG	serosanguineous	SGD	straight gravity drainage
		SGE	significant glandular enlargement
SERs	somatosensory evoked responses	s̄ gl	without correction/ without glasses
SES	socioeconomic status		
SEWHO	shoulder-elbow-wrist-hand orthosis	SGM	serum glucose monitoring
SF	salt free	SGOT	serum glutamic oxaloacetic transaminase (same as AST)
	saturated fat		
	scarlet fever		
	seizure frequency	SGPT	serum glutamic pyruvic transaminase (same as ALT)
	seminal fluid		
	soft feces		
	sound field	SGS	second-generation sulfonylurea
	spinal fluid		

	subglottic stenosis	SIDS	sudden infant death syndrome
SH	serum hepatitis		
	short	SIEP	serum immunoelectro-phoresis
	shoulder		
	shower	Sig.	let it be marked (appears on prescription before directions for patient)
	social history		
	surgical history		
S&H	speech and hearing	SIJ	sacroiliac joint
S/H	suicidal/homicidal ideation	SIL	sister-in-law
		SILFVD	sterile indicated low forceps vaginal delivery
SHA	super heated aerosol		
SHAL	standard hyperalimenta-tion	SILV	simultaneous independent lung ventilation
S Hb	sickle hemoglobin screen	SIM	selective ion monitoring
SHBG	serum hormone-binding globulin		Similac®
		Sim c̄ Fe	Similac with iron®
SHEENT	skin, head, eyes, ears, nose, and throat	SIMV	synchronized intermittent mandatory ventilation
SHI	standard heparin infusion	SIP	Sickness Impact Profile
Shig	*Shigella*	SIS	sister
SHL	supraglottic horizontal laryngectomy		Surgical Infection Stratification (system)
SHS	student health service	SISI	short increment sensitivity index
SI	International System of Units		
		SISS	severe invasion streptococcal syndrome
	sacroiliac		
	sector iridectomy	SIT	silicon-intensified target
	self-inflicted		Slossen Intelligence Test
	seriously ill		sperm immobilization test
	small intestine		surgical intensive therapy
	strict isolation	SIT BAL	sitting balance
	stress incontinence	SIT TOL	sitting tolerance
	stroke index	SIV	simian immunodeficiency virus
	suicidal ideation		
SIADH	syndrome of inappropriate antidiuretic hormone secretion	SIVP	slow intravenous push
		SIW	self-inflicted wound
		SJS	Stevens-Johnson syndrome
S & I	suction and irrigation		
SIB	self-injurious behavior		Swyer-James syndrome
sibs	siblings	SK	seborrheic keratosis
SICT	selective intracoronary thrombolysis		senile keratosis
			SmithKline®
SICU	surgical intensive care unit		solar keratosis
SIDA	French and Spanish abbreviation for AIDS		streptokinase
		SKAO	supracondylar knee-ankle orthosis
SIDD	syndrome of isolated diastolic dysfunction		
		SK-SD	streptokinase streptodornase
SIDFF	superimposed dorsiflexion of foot		
		SL	sensation level

	shortleg		urination, and
	slight		defecation
	sublingual	SLV	since last visit
S/L	slit lamp (examination)	SLWB	severely low birth weight
SLA	sacrolaeva anterior	SLWC	short leg walking cast
	sex and love addictions	SM	sadomasochism
	slide latex agglutination		skim milk
SLAA	Sex and Love Addicts		small
	Anonymous		Stairmaster®
SLAC	scapholunate advanced		streptomycin
	collapse		systolic murmur
SLAP	serum leucine	SMA	sequential multiple
	amino-peptidase		analyzer
SLB	short leg brace		simultaneous multichannel
SLC	short leg cast		auto-analyzer
SLCC	short leg cylinder cast		spinal muscular atrophy
SLCT	Sertoli-Leydig cell tumor		superior mesenteric artery
SLE	slit lamp examination	SMA-6	sequential multipler
	St. Louis encephalitis		analyzer for sodium,
	systemic lupus		potassium, CO_2,
	erythematosus		chloride, glucose, and
SLFVD	sterile low forceps vaginal		BUN
	delivery	SMA-7	sodium, potassium, CO_2,
SLGXT	symptom limited graded		chloride, glucose,
	exercise test		BUN, and creatinine
SLK	superior limbic	SMA-12	glucose, BUN, uric acid,
	keratoconjunctivitis		calcium, phosphorus,
SLL	small lymphocytic		total protein, albumin,
	lymphoma		cholesterol, total
SLMFVD	sterile low mid-forceps		bilirubin, alkaline
	vaginal delivery		phosphatase, SGOT,
SLMP	since last menstrual		and LDH
	period	SMA-23	includes the entire
SLN	superior laryngeal nerve		SMA-12 plus sodium,
SLNTG	sublingual nitroglycerin		potassium, CO_2,
SLNWBC	short leg nonweight-		chloride, direct
	bearing cast		bilirubin, triglyceride,
SLNWC	short leg non-walking cast		SGPT, indirect
SLO	streptolysin O		bilirubin, R fraction,
SLP	speech language		and BUN/creatinine
	pathology		ratio
SLR	straight leg raising	SMAS	superficial musculoapo-
SLRT	straight leg raising test		neurotic system
SLS	short leg splint	SMBG	self-monitoring blood
	single limb support		glucose
SLT	swing light test	SMC	special mouth care
SLT	sacrolaeva transversa	SMCD	senile macular
sl. tr.	slight trace		chorioretinal
SLUD	salivation, lacrimation,		degeneration

SMD	senile macular degeneration		Student Nursing Assistant
		SNAP	sensory nerve action potential
SMF	streptozocin, mitomycin, and fluorouracil	SNAT	suspected non-accidental trauma
SMFVD	sterile mid-forceps vaginal delivery	SNB	scalene node biopsy
SMI	safety, monitoring, intervention, length of stay and evaluation	SNC	skilled nursing care
		SNCV	sensory nerve conduction velocity
	sensory motor integration (group)	SND	single needle device sinus node dysfunction
	severely mentally impaired	SNE	subacute necrotizing encephalomyelopathy
	small volume infusion	SNEP	student nurse extern program
	suggested minimum increment	SNF	skilled nursing facility
	sustained maximal inspiration	SNGFR	single nephron glomerular filtration rate
SMILE	sustained maximal inspiratory lung exercises	SNHL	sensorineural hearing loss
		SNIP	strict no information in paper
SMO	Senior Medical Officer slip made out	SNOOP	Systematic Nursing Observation of Psychopathology
SMON	subacute myelo-opticoneuropathy	SNP	simple neonatal procedure sodium nitroprusside
SMP	self-management program		
SMPN	sensorimotor polyneuropathy	SNR	signal-to-noise ratio
		SNRT	sinus node recovery time
SMR	senior medical resident skeletal muscle relaxant	SNS	sterile normal saline (0.9% sodium chloride)
	standardized mortality ratio	SNT	sinuses, nose, and throat suppan nail technique
	submucosal resection	SO	second opinion
SMRR	submucous resection and rhinoplasty		shoulder orthosis
			significant other
SMS	senior medical student somatostatin		sphincter of Oddi
			standing orders
SMV	submentovertical superior mesenteric vein		suboccipital
			superior oblique
SMVT	sustained monomorphic ventricular tachycardia		supraoptic
			supraorbital
SMX-TMP	sulfamethoxazole and trimethoprim		sutures out
		S-O	salpingo-oophorectomy
SN	sciatic notch	S&O	salpingo-oophorectomy
	student nurse	SO₃	sulfite
	superior nasal	SO₄	sulfate
Sn	tin	SOA	serum opsonic activity
S/N	signal to noise ratio		spinal opioid analgesia
SNA	specimen not available		supraorbital artery

	swelling of ankles	SP	sacrum to pubis
SOAA	signed out against advice		semiprivate
SOAM	sutures out in the morning		sequential pulse
SOAMA	signed out against medical advice		spastic dysphonia
			speech
SOAP	subjective, objective, assessment, and plans		Speech Pathologist
			spouse
SOAPIE	subjective, objective, assessment, plan, intervention, and evaluation		stand pivot
			suicide precautions
			suprapubic
		sp	species
SOB	see order book	S/P	semiprivate
	shortness of breath (this abbreviation has caused problems)		serum protein
			shoulder press
			spinal
	side of bed		stand and pivot
SOC	socialization		status post
	standard of care		suicide precautions
	state of consciousness		suprapubic
S & OC	signed and on chart (e.g. permit)		systolic pressure
		SP 1	suicide precautions number 1
SOD	sinovenous occlusive disease	SP 2	suicide precautions number 2
	superoxide dysmutase		
	surgical officer of the day	SPA	albumin human (formerly known as salt-poor albumin)
SODAS	spheriodal oral drug absorption system		
			serum prothrombin activity
SOG	suggestive of good		single photon absorptiometry
SOI	syrup of ipecac		
SOL	solution		stimulation produced analgesia
	space occupying lesion		
SOM	serous otitis media		student physician's assistant
SOMI	sterno-occipital mandibular immobilizer		
			suprapubic aspiration
Sono	sonogram	SPAC	satisfactory postanesthesia course
SONP	solid organs not palpable		
SOP	standard operating procedure	SPAG	small particle aerosol generator
SOPM	stitches out in afternoon		
SOR	sign own release	SPAMM	spatial modulation of magnetization
SOS	if there is need		
	may be repeated once if urgently required (Latin: *si opus sit*)	SPBI	serum protein bound iodine
		SPBT	suprapubic bladder tap
	self-obtained smear	SPC	suprapubic catheter
SOSOB	sit on side of bed	SPCT	simultaneous prism and cover test
SOT	something other than		
	stream of thought	SPD	subcorneal pustular dermatosis
	superficial ocular trauma		

Supply, Processing, and Distribution (department)

suprapubic drainage

SPET single-photon emission tomography

SPE serum protein electrophoresis

SPEC specimen

SPECT single photon emission computer tomography

Spec Ed special education

SPEEP spontaneous positive end-expiratory pressure

SPEP serum protein electrophoresis

SPET single-photon emission tomography

SPF split products of fibrin
sun protective factor

sp fl spinal fluid

SPG scrotopenogram
sphenopalatine ganglion

Sp.G specific gravity

SPH spherocytes

SPHERO spherocytes

SPI speech processor interface
surgical peripheral iridectomy

SPIA solid phase immunoabsorbent assay

SPIF spontaneous peak inspiratory force

SPL sound pressure level

SPK superficial punctate keratitis

SPMA spinal progressive muscle atrophy

SPMSQ Short Portable Mental Status Questionnaire

SPN solitary pulmonary nodule
student practical nurse

SPO status postoperative

spont spontaneous

SPP species (specus)
super packed platelets
suprapubic prostatectomy

SPRAS Sheehan Patient Rated Anxiety Scale

SPROM spontaneous premature rupture of membrane

SPS simple partial seizure
sodium polyethanol sulfonate
sodium polystyrene sulfonate
systemic progressive sclerosis

SPT skin prick test

SP TAP spinal tap

SP TUBE suprapubic tube

SPTX static pelvic traction

SPU short procedure unit

SPVR systemic peripheral vascular resistance

SQ status quo
subcutaneous (this is a dangerous abbreviation)

Sq CCa squamous cell carcinoma

SR screen
sedimentation rate
side rails
sinus rhythm
smooth-rough
sustained release
suture removal
system review

S&R seclusion and restraint

SRBC sheep red blood cells
sickle red blood cells

SRBOW spontaneous rupture of bag of waters

SRD service-related disability
sodium-restricted diet

SRF somatotropin releasing factor
subretinal fluid

SRF-A slow releasing factor of anaphylaxis

SRH signs of recent hemorrhage

SRI serotonin re-uptake inhibitor

SRICU surgical respiratory intensive care unit

SRIF somatotropin-

	release inhibiting factor (somatostatin)	S&S	shower and shampoo
			signs and symptoms
SRMD	stress-related mucosal damage		sling and swathe
SR/NE	sinus rhythm, no ectopy		support and stimulation
SRNVM	senile retinal neovascular membrane		swish and spit
			swish and swallow
	subretinal neovascular membrane	SSA	sagittal split advancement
			salicylsalicylic acid (salsalate)
SRO	single room occupancy		Sjögren's syndrome antigen A
SROCPI	Self-Rating Obsessive-Compulsive Personality Inventory		Social Security Administration
SROM	spontaneous rupture of membrane		sulfasalicylic acid (test)
SRP	septorhinoplasty	SSC	sign symptom complex
	stapes replacement prosthesis		Special Services for Children
S̄R̄S̄	without redness or swelling	SSc	systemic sclerosis
SRS-A	slow-reacting substance of anaphylaxis	SSCA	single shoulder contrast arthrography
SRT	sedimentation rate test	SSCP	substernal chest pain
	sleep-related tumescence	SSCr	stainless steel crown
	speech reception threshold	SSCU	surgical special care unit
	surfactant replacement therapy	SSCVD	sterile spontaneous controlled vaginal delivery
	sustained release theophylline	SSD	serosanguineous drainage
SRU	side rails up		sickle cell disease
SRUS	solitary rectal ulcer syndrome		silver sulfadiazine
			Social Security disability
			source to skin distance
SR ⚡X2	both siderails up	SSDI	Social Security disability income
SS	half	SSE	saline solution enema
	sacrosciatic		soapsuds enema
	saline solution		systemic side effects
	saliva sample	SSEPs	somatosensory evoked potentials
	salt substitute	SSF	subscapular skinfold
	sickle cell	SSG	sublabial salivary gland
	Sjögren's syndrome	SSI	sub-shock insulin
	sliding scale		Supplemental Security Income
	slip sent		
	Social Security	SSKI	saturated solution of potassium iodide
	social service		
	somatostatin	SSL	subtotal supraglottic laryngectomy
	steady state		
	susceptible	SSM	superficial spreading melanoma
	suprasciatic (notch)		
	symmetrical strength		

SSN	Social Security number	stab.	polymorphonuclear leukocytes (white blood cells, in nonmature form)
SSO	short stay observation (unit)		
	Spanish speaking only		
SSOP	Second Surgical Opinion Program	STAI	State-Trait Anxiety Inventory
SSP	short stay procedure (unit)	STAI-I	State-Trait-Anxiety Index—I
SSPE	subacute sclerosing panencephalitis	STA-MCA	superficial temporary artery-middle cerebral artery (bypass)
SSPL	saturation sound pressure level		
SSPU	surgical short procedure unit	STAPES	stapedectomy
		staph	*Staphylococcus aureus*
SSR	substernal retractions	stat	immediately
	sympathetic skin response	STB	stillborn
SSRI	selective serotonin reuptake inhibitor	STBAL	standing balance
		ST BY	stand by
SSS	layer upon layer	STC	serum theophylline concentration
	scalded skin syndrome		soft tissue calcification
	Sepsis Severity Score		stimulate to cry
	short stay service (unit)		subtotal colectomy
	sick sinus syndrome		sugar tongue cast
	skin and skin structures	ST CLK	station clerk
	sterile saline soak	STD	sexually transmitted diseases
SSSB	sagittal split setback		
SSSIs	skin and skin structure infections		skin test dose
			skin to tumor distance
SSSS	staphylococcal scalded skin syndrome		sodium tetradecyl sulfate
		STD TF	standard tube feeding
SST	sagittal sinus thrombosis	STEAM	stimulated-echo acquisition mode
SSX	sulfisoxazole acetyl		
S/SX	signs/symptoms	STET	single photon emission tomography
ST	esotropic		
	sacrum transverse		submaximal treadmill exercise test
	shock therapy		
	sinus tachycardia	STETH	stethoscope
	skin test	STF	special tube feeding
	slight trace		standard tube feeding
	speech therapist	STG	short-term goals
	speech therapy		split-thickness graft
	split thickness	STH	soft tissue hemorrhage
	stomach		somatotrophic hormone
	straight		subtotal hysterectomy
	stress testing		supplemental thyroid hormone
	stretcher		
	subtotal	STHB	said to have been
	Surgical Technologist	STI	soft tissue injury
STA	second trimester abortion	STILLB	stillborn
	superficial temporal artery		

STIR	short TI inversion recovery	S/U	shoulder/umbilicus
STIs	systolic time intervals	SUA	serum uric acid
STJ	subtalar joint		single umbilical artery
STK	streptokinase	SUB	Skene's urethra and Bartholin's glands
STL	serum theophylline level		
STLE	St. Louis encephalitis	SUBL	sublingual
STLOM	swelling, tenderness, and limitation of motion	Subcu	subcutaneous
		SUB-MAND	submandibular
STM	short-term memory streptomycin	sub q	subcutaneous (this is a dangerous abbreviation since the q is mistaken for every, when a number follows)
STMT	Seat Movement		
STNM	surgical evaluative staging of cancer		
STNR	symmetrical tonic neck reflex	SUD	sudden unexpected death
		SUDS	Subjective Unit of Distress (Disturbance) (discomfort) Scale
STOP	sensitive, timely, and organized programs (battered spouses)		
		SUI	stress urinary incontinence
STORCH	syphilis, toxoplasmosis, other agents, rubella, cytomegalovirus, and herpes (maternal infections)		suicide
		SUID	sudden unexplained infant death
		SULF-PRIM	trimethoprim and sulfamethoxazole
STP	short-term plans sodium thiopental	SUN	serum urea nitrogen
STPD	standard temperature and pressure—dry	SUNDS	sudden unexplained nocturnal death syndrome
STR	stretcher		
strep	streptococcus streptomycin	SUP	superior supination supinator symptomatic uterine prolapse
STS	serologic test for syphilis sodium tetradecyl sulfate soft tissue swelling Surgical Technology Student		
		supp	suppository
		SUR	surgery; surgical
STSG	split thickness skin graft	Surgi	Surgigator
STT	scaphoid, trapezium trapezoid skin temperature test	SUUD	sudden unexpected, unexplained death
		SUX	succinylcholine suction
STTOL	standing tolerance		
STU	shock trauma unit surgical trauma unit	SV	seminal vesical sigmoid volvulus single ventricle stock volume
STV	short-term variability		
STX	stricture		
STZ	streptozocin	SVA	small volume admixture
S&U	supine and upright	SVB	saphenous vein bypass
SU	sensory urgency Somogyi units	SVC	slow vital capacity superior vena cava

SVCO	superior vena cava obstruction		SWT	stab wound of the throat
			SWU	septic work-up
SVCS	superior vena cava syndrome		Sx	signs
				surgery
SVD	single vessel disease			symptom
	spontaneous vaginal delivery		SXR	skull x-ray
			syr	syrup
SVE	sterile vaginal examination		SYS BP	systolic blood pressure
			SZ	schizophrenic
	Streptococcus viridans endocarditis			seizure
				suction
SV&E	suicidal, violent, and eloper		SZN	streptozocin
SVG	saphenous vein graft			
SVL	severe visual loss			
SVN	small volume nebulizer			

T

SVO$_2$	mixed venous oxygen saturation			
SVP	spontaneous venous pulse		T	tablespoon (15 mL) (this is a dangerous abbreviation)
SVPB	supraventricular premature beat			
SVPC	supraventricular premature contraction			temperature
				tender
SVR	supraventricular rhythm			tension
	systemic vascular resistance			testicles
				thoracic
SVRI	systemic vascular resistance index			trace
SVT	supraventricular tachycardia		t	teaspoon (5 mL) (this is a dangerous abbreviation)
SVVD	spontaneous vertex vaginal delivery		T+	increase tension
SW	sandwich		T-	decreased tension
	Social Worker		T$_{1/2}$	half-life
	stab wound		T$_1$	tricuspid first sound
S&W	soap and water		T-2	dactinomycin, doxorubicin, vincristine, and cyclophosphamide
S/W	somewhat			
SWD	short wave diathermy			
SWFI	sterile water for injection			
SWG	standard wire gauge		T$_3$	triiodothyronine
SWI	sterile water for injection		T3	Tylenol® with codeine 30 mg (this is a dangerous abbreviation)
	surgical wound infection			
S&WI	skin and wound isolation			
SWOG	Southwest Oncology Group		T$_4$	levothyroxine
				thyroxine
SWP	small whirlpool		T$_{3/4}$ind	triiodothyronine to thyroxine index
SWS	slow wave sleep			
	student ward secretary			
	Sturge-Weber syndrome		T-7	free thyroxine factor

167

$T_1...T_{12}$	thoracic nerve 1 through 12		total arm length
		T ALCON	Alcon® tonometry
	thoracic vertebra 1 through 12	TAML	therapy-related acute myelogenous leukemia
TA	Takayasu's arteritis	TAM	tamoxifen
	temperature axillary		teenage mother
	temporal arteritis	TAN	Treatment Authorization Number
	therapeutic abortion		
	tracheal aspirate		tropical ataxic neuropathy
	traffic accident	TANI	total axial (lymph) node irradiation
	tricuspid atresia		
Ta	tonometry applanation	TAO	thromboangitis obliterans
T&A	tonsillectomy and adenoidectomy		troleandomycin
		TAP	tonometry by applanation
T(A)	axillary temperature	T APPL	applanation tonometry
TAA	thoracic aortic aneurysm	TAPVC	total anomalous pulmonary venous connection
	total ankle arthroplasty		
	transverse aortic arch		
	triamcinolone acetonide	TAPVD	total anomalous pulmonary venous drainage
	tumor associated antigen (antibodies)		
TAB	tablet	TAPVR	total anomalous pulmonary venous return
	therapeutic abortion		
	triple antibiotic (bacitracin, neomycin, and polymyxin—this is a dangerous abbreviation)	TAR	thrombocytopenia with absent radius
			total ankle replacement
			treatment authorization request
TAC	tetracaine, Adrenalin® and cocaine	TARA	total articular replacement arthroplasty
	tibial artery catheter	TAS	therapeutic activities specialist
	triamicinolone cream		
TAD	transverse abdominal diameter		typical absence seizures
TADAC	therapeutic abortion, dilation, aspiration, and curettage	TAT	tetanus antitoxin
			till all taken
			thematic apperception test
TAE	transcatheter arterial embolization	TB	terrible burning
			toothbrush
TAF	tissue angiogenesis factor		total base
TAH	total abdominal hysterectomy		total bilirubin
			total body
	total artificial heart		tuberculosis
TAHBSO	total abdominal hysterectomy, bilateral salpingo-oophorectomy	TBA	to be absorbed
			to be added
			to be admitted
T Air	air puff tonometry		total body (surface) area
TAL	tendon Achilles lengthening	TBB	transbronchial biopsy
		TBC	total blood cholesterol

	total body clearance	Tc	technetium
	tuberculosis	T/C	telephone call
TBE	tick-born encephalitis		to consider
TBF	total body fat	TC7	Interceed®
TBG	thyroxine-binding globulin	T&C	turn and cough
			type and crossmatch
TBI	toothbrushing instruction	T&C#3	Tylenol® with 30 mg codeine
	total body irradiation		
	traumatic brain injury	TCA	team conference
T bili	total bilirubin		terminal cancer
TBK	total body potassium		thioguanine and cytarabine
tbl.	tablespoon (15 mL)		trichloroacetic acid
TBLB	transbronchial lung biopsy		tricuspid atresia
TBLC	term birth, living child		tricyclic antidepressant
TBLF	term birth, living female	TCABG	triple coronary artery bypass graft
TBLM	term birth, living male		
TBM	tracheobronchomalacia	TCAD	tricyclic antidepressant
	tubule basement membrane	TCAR	tiazofurin
TBNA	total body sodium	TCBS agar	thiosulfate-citrate-bile salt-sucrose agar
	transbronchial needle aspiration		
	treated but not admitted	TCC	transitional cell carcinoma
TBOCS	Tale-Brown Obsessive-Compulsive Scale	TCD	transcerebellar diameter
			transverse cardiac diameter
TBP	total-body photographs	TCCB	transitional cell carcinoma of bladder
TBPA	thyroxine-binding prealbumin		
		TCDB	turn, cough, and deep breath
TBR	total bed rest		
TBSA	total body surface area	TCDD	tetrachlorodibenzo-p-dioxin
	total burn surface area		
tbsp	tablespoon (15 mL)	99mTc DTPA	technetium Tc 99m pentetate
TBT	tolbutamide test		
	tracheal bronchial toilet	TCE	tetrachloroethylene
	transbronchoscopic balloon tipped	T cell	small lymphocyte
		99mTcGHA	technetium Tc 99m gluceptate
TBV	total blood volume		
	transluminal balloon valvuloplasty	TCH	turn, cough, hyperventilate
TBW	total body water	TCID	tissue culture infective dose
TBX®	thiabendazole		
TC	thoracic circumference	TCL	tibial collateral ligament
	throat culture	TCM	tissue culture media
	tissue culture		traditional Chinese medicine
	total cholesterol		transcutaneous (oxygen) monitor
	to (the) chest		
	trauma center	99mTc-	technetium Tc 99m
	true conjugate		
	tubocurarine		

MAA	albumin microaggregated	TDF	testis determining factor
			tumor dose fractionation
TCMH	tumor-direct cell-mediated hypersensitivity	TDI	toluene diisocyanate
		TDK	tardive diskinesia
TCMS	transcranial cortical magnetic stimulation	TDL	thoracic duct lymph
		TDM	therapeutic drug monitoring
TCMZ	trichloromethiazide		
TCN	tetracycline	TDMAC	tridodecylmethyl ammonium chloride
	triciribine phosphate (tricyclic nucleoside)		
		TDN	transdermal nitroglycerin
TCNS	transcutaneous nerve stimulator	TDNTG	transdermal nitroglycerin
		TdP	torsades de pointes
TCNU	tauromustine	TdR	thymidine
TcO_4^-	pertechnetate	TDT	tentative discharge tomorrow
TCOM	transcutaneous oxygen monitor		
		TdT	terminal deoxynucleotidyl transferase
TCP	tranylcypromine		
$TcPCO_2$	transcutaneous carbon dioxide	TDWB	touch down weight bearing
$TcPO_2$	transcutaneous oxygen	$TDx^®$	fluorescence polarization immunoassay
$^{99m}TcPYP$	technetium Tc 99m pyrophosphate		
		TE	echo time
TCR	T-cell receptor		tennis elbow
TCRE	transcervical resection of the endometrium		tooth extraction
			trace elements
$^{99m}TcSC$	technetium Tc 99m sulfur colloid		tracheoesophageal
			transesophageal echocardiography
TCT	thyrocalcitonin		
	tincture	T&E	trial and error
TCU	transitional care unit	TEA	thromboendarterectomy
TCVA	thromboembolic cerebral vascular accident		total elbow arthroplasty
		TEC	total eosinophil count
TD	Takayasu's disease	T&EC	trauma and emergency center
	tardive dyskinesia		
	tetanus-diphtheria toxoid (pediatric use)	$TEDS^®$	anti-embolism stockings
		TEE	transesophageal echocardiography
	tidal volume		
	tone decay	TEF	tracheoesophageal fistula
	total disability	TEG	thromboelastogram
	transverse diameter	TEI	total episode of illness
	travelers' diarrhea		transesophageal imaging
	treatment discontinued	TEL	telemetry
Td	tetanus-diphtheria toxoid (adult type)	tele	telemetry
		TEM	transmission electron microscopy
TDD	telephone device for the deaf		
		TEN	tension (intraocular pressure)
	thoracic duct drainage		
TDE	total daily energy (requirement)		toxic epidermal necrolysis
		$TEN^®$	Total Enteral Nutrition

TENS	transcutaneous electrical nerve stimulation	TGXT	thallium-graded exercise test
TEP	tracheoesophageal puncture	TH	thrill
	tubal ectopic pregnancy		thyroid hormone
TER	total elbow replacement		total hysterectomy
	total energy requirement	T&H	type and hold
	transurethral electroresection	THA	tacrine (tetrahydroacridine)
			total hip arthroplasty
TERB	terbutaline		transient hemispheric attack
tert.	tertiary	THBR	thyroid hormone-binding ratio
TES	treatment emergent symptoms	THAM®	tromethamine
TESS	Treatment Emergent Symptom Scale	THC	tetrahydrocannabinol (dronabinol)
TET	transcranial electrostimulation therapy		transhepatic cholangiogram
	treadmill exercise test	TH-CULT	throat culture
TEV	talipes equinovarus (deformity)	THE	transhepatic embolization
TF	tactile fremitus	Ther Ex	therapeutic exercise
	tetralogy of Fallot	THF	thymic humoral factor
	to follow	THI	transient hypogammaglobinemia of infancy
	tube feeding	THKAFO	trunk-hip-knee-ankle-foot orthosis
TFB	trifascicular block		
TFF	tangential flow filtration	THP	take home packs
TFL	tensor fasciae latae		transhepatic portography
TFM	transverse friction massage		trihexyphenidyl
TFT	trifluridine (trifluorothymidine)	THR	total hip replacement
			training heart rate
TFTs	thyroid function tests	THTV	therapeutic home trial visit
TG	triglycerides	TI	terminal ileus
6-TG	thioguanine		transischial
TGA	transient global amnesia		tricuspid insufficiency
	transposition of the great arteries	TIA	transient ischemic attack
		tib.	tibia
TGFA	triglyceride fatty acid	TIBC	total iron-binding capacity
TGF	transforming growth factor	TIC	trypsin-inhibitor capacity
TGF-β	transforming growth factor-beta	TICU	transplant intensive care unit
			trauma intensive care unit
TGGE	temperature-gradient gel electrophoresis	TID	three times a day
TGS	tincture of green soap	TIDM	three times daily with meals
TGs	triglycerides	TIE	transient ischemic episode
TGT	thromboplastin generation test	TIG	tetanus immune globulin
TGV	thoracic gas volume	TIL	tumor-infiltrating lymphocytes

%tile	percentile		total lung capacity
TIMP	tissue inhibitor of metalloproteinase		total lymphocyte count
			triple lumen catheter
TIN	three times a night (this is a dangerous abbreviation)	TLD	thermoluminescent dosimeter
		TLE	temporal lobe epilepsy
tinct	tincture	TLI	total lymphoid irradiation
TIPS	transjugular intrahepatic portosystemic shunt		translaryngeal intubation
		TLK	thermal laser keratoplasty
TIS	tumor *in situ*	TLNB	term living newborn
TISS	Therapeutic Intervention Scoring System	TLP	transitional living program
		TLR	tonic labyrinthine reflex
TIT	*Treponema (pallidum)* immobilization test	TLS	tumor lysis syndrome
		TLSO	thoracic lumbar sacral orthosis
	triiodothyronine		
TIUP	term intrauterine pregnancy	TLSSO	thoracolumbosacral spinal orthosis
TIVC	thoracic inferior vena cava	TLT	tonsillectomy
		TLV	total lung volume
+tive	positive	TM	temperature by mouth
TIW	three times a week (this is a dangerous abbreviation)		Thayer-Martin (culture)
			trabecular meshwork
			transcendental meditation
TJ	triceps jerk		treadmill
TJA	total joint arthroplasty		tumor
TJN	twin jet nebulizer		tympanic membrane
TK	thymidine kinase	T & M	type and crossmatch
TKA	total knee arthroplasty	TMA	thrombotic microangiopathy
TKD	tokodynamometer		
TKE	terminal knee extension		transmetatarsal amputation
TKNO	to keep needle open		
TKP	thermokeratoplasty	T/MA	tracheostomy mask
TKO	to keep open	TMAS	Taylor Manifest Anxiety Scale
TKR	total knee replacement		
TKVO	to keep vein open	T_{max}	temperature maximum
TL	team leader	t_{max}	time of occurrence for maximum (peak) drug concentration
	transverse line		
	trial leave		
	tubal ligation	TMB	transient monocular blindness
T/L	terminal latency		
Tl	thallium		trimethoxybenzoates
TLA	translumbar arteriogram (aortogram)	TMC	transmural colitis
			triamcinolone
TLAC	triple lumen arrow catheter	TMCA	trimethylcolchicinic acid
		TME	thermolysin-like metalloendopeptidase
TLC	tender loving care		
	thin layer chromatography	TMET	tread mill exercise test
	T-lymphocyte choriocarcinoma	TMI	threatened myocardial infarction

172

TMJ	temporomandibular joint	T(O)	oral temperature
TML	treadmill	T&O	tubes and ovaries
TMM	torn medial meniscus	TOA	time of arrival
	total muscle mass		tubo-ovarian abscess
Tmm	McKay-Marg tension	TOB	tobacco
TMNG	toxic multinodular goiter		tobramycin
TMP	thallium myocardial	TOC	total organic carbon
	perfusion	TOCE	transcatheter oily
	transmembrane pressure		chemoembolization
	trimethoprim	TOCO	tocodynamometer
TMP/SMX	trimethoprim and	TOD	intraocular pressure of the
	sulfamethoxazole		right eye
TMR	trainable mentally	TOF	tetralogy of Fallot
	retarded		total of four
TMST	treadmill stress test		train-of-four
TMT	treadmill test	TOGV	transposition of the great
TMTC	too many to count		vessels
TMTX	trimetrexate	TOH	throughout hospitalization
TM-WKTM	tender mass with known tissue malignancy	TOL	tolerate trial of labor
TMX	tamoxifen	TOM	tomorrow
TMZ	temazepam		transcutaneous oxygen
TN	normal intraocular tension		monitor
	team nursing	Tomo	tomography
	temperature normal	TON	tonight
T&N	tension and nervousness	TOP	termination of pregnancy
TNA	total nutrient admixture	TOPV	trivalent oral polio
TNB	term newborn		vaccine
	Tru-Cut® needle biopsy	TORCH	toxoplasmosis, other
TNBP	transurethral needle		(syphillis, hepatitis,
	biopsy of prostate		zoster), rubella, cytome-
TNF	tumor necrosis factor		galovirus, and herpes
TNG	nitroglycerin		simplex (maternal
TNI	total nodal irradiation		infections)
TNM	primary tumor, regional	TORP	total ossicular
	lymph nodes, and		replacement prosthesis
	distant metastasis (used	TOS	intraocular pressure of the
	with subscripts for the		left eye
	staging of cancer)		thoracic outlet syndrome
TNS	transcutaneous nerve	TOT BILI	total bilirubin
	stimulation (stimulator)	TP	temperature and pressure
	Tullie-Niebörg syndrome		temporoparietal
TNT	triamcinolone and nystatin		therapeutic pass
TNTC	too numerous to count		thrombophlebitis
TO	old tuberculin		Todd's paralysis
	telephone order		total protein
	time off		"T" piece
	total obstruction		treating physician
	transfer out	T & P	temperature and pulse

	turn and position		transfusion reaction
			transplant recipients
TPA	alteplase, recombinant (tissue plasminogen activator)		treatment
			tremor
	tissue polypeptide antigen		tricuspid regurgitation
	total parenteral alimentation		tumor registry
		T(R)	rectal temperature
TPC	total patient care	T & R	tenderness and rebound
TPD	tropical pancreatic diabetes	TRA	therapeutic recreation associate
TPE	therapeutic plasma exchange		to run at
		trach.	tracheal
	total protective environment		tracheostomy
TPF	trained participating father	TRAFO	tone-reducing ankle/foot orthosis
TPH	thromboembolic pulmonary hypertension	Trans D	transverse diameter
		TRAP	tartrate-resistant (leukocyte) acid phophatase
	trained participating husband		
T PHOS	triple phosphate crystals		trapezium
TPI	*Treponema pallidum* immobilization	TRAS	transplant renal artery stenosis
TPL	thromboplastin	TRC	tanned red cells
T plasty	tympanoplasty	TRD	tongue-retaining device
TPM	temporary pacemaker		traction retinal detachment
TPN	total parenteral nutrition		
TP & P	time, place, and person	Tren	Trendelenburg
TPO	thrombopoietin	TRH	protirelin (thyrotropin-releasing hormone)
	trial prescription order		
TPP	thiamine pyrophosphate	TRI	trimester
TPPN	total peripheral parenteral nutrition	T_3RIA	triiodothyronine level by radioimmunoassay
TPPV	trans pars plana vitrectomy	TRIC	trachoma inclusion conjunctivitis
TPR	temperature	TRICH	*Trichomonas*
	temperature, pulse, and respiration	TRIG	triglycerides
		TRISS	Trauma Score and Injury Severity Score
	total peripheral resistance		
T PROT	total protein	TR-LSC	time-resolved liquid scintillation counting
TPT	time to peak tension		
	transpyloric tube	TRM-SMX	trimethoprim-sulfamethoxazole
	treadmill performance test		
TPU	tropical phagedenic ulcer	tRNA	transfer ribonucleic acid
TPVR	total peripheral vascular resistance	TRND	Trendelenburg
		TRNG	tetracycline-resistant *Neisseria gonorrhoeae*
TR	therapeutic recreation		
	tincture	TRO	to return to office
	to return	TRP	tubular reabsorption of phosphate
	trace		

TRPT	transplant	T-SKULL	trauma skull
TRS	Therapeutic Recreation Specialist	tsp	teaspoon (5 mL)
		TSP	total serum protein
	the real symptom		tropical spastic paraparesis
TRT	thermoradiotherapy		
TR/TE	time to repetition and time to echo in spin (echo sequence of magnetic resonance imaging)	TSPA	thiotepa
		T-SPINE	thoracic spine
		TSR	total shoulder replacement
		TSS	toxic shock syndrome
		TST	titmus stereocuity test
T_3RU	triiodothyronine resin uptake		trans-scrotal testosterone
			treadmill stress test
TRUS	transrectal ultrasound		tuberculin skin test(s)
TRUSP	transrectal ultrasound of the prostate	TSTA	tumor-specific transplantation antigens
TRZ	triazolam	T&T	tobramycin and ticarcillin
TS	temperature sensitive		touch and tone
	test solution	TT	Test Tape®
	thoracic spine		tetanus toxoid
	toe signs		thrombin time
	Tourette's syndrome		thymol turbidity
	transsexual		tilt table
	Trauma Score		tonometry
	tricuspid stenosis		transtracheal
	triple strength		twitch tension
	Turner's syndrome		tympanic temperature
T&S	type and screen	T/T	trace of ___ /trace of___
Ts	Schiotz tension	TT4	total thyroxine
TSAb	thyroid stimulating antibodies	TTA	total toe arthroplasty
		TTC	transtracheal catheter
TSA	toluenesulfonic acid	TTD	temporary total disability
	total shoulder arthroplasty		transverse thoracic diameter
TSAR®	tape surrounded Appli-rulers	TTE	transthoracic echocardiography
TSB	trypticase soy broth		
TSBB	transtracheal selective bronchial brushing	TTM	total tumor mass
		TTN	transient tachypnea of the newborn
TSC	technetium sulfur colloid		
	theophylline serum concentration	TTNA	transthoracic needle aspiration
TSD	target to skin distance	TTNB	transient tachypnea of the newborn
	Tay-Sachs disease		
TSE	targeted systemic exposure	TTO	to take out
			transtracheal oxygen
T set	tracheotomy set	TTOD	tetanus toxoid outdated
TSE	testicular self-examination	TTOT	transtracheal oxygen therapy
TSF	tricep skin fold		
TSH	thyroid-stimulating hormone	TTP	thrombotic thrombocy-topenic purpura

175

TTR	triceps tendon reflex		*Trichomonas vaginalis*
TTS	tarsal tunnel syndrome	T/V	touch-verbal
	temporary threshold shift	TVC	triple voiding cystogram
	through the skin		true vocal cord
	transdermal therapeutic system	TVD	triple vessel disease
	transfusion therapy service	TVDALV	triple vessel disease with an abnormal left ventricle
TTT	tilt table test	TVF	tactile vocal fremitus
	tolbutamide tolerance test	TVH	total vaginal hysterectomy
TTUTD	tetanus toxoid up-to-date	TVN	tonic vibration response
TTVP	temporary transvenous pacemaker	TVP	transvenous pacemaker transvesicle prostatectomy
TTWB	touch toe weight bearing	TVR	tricuspid valve replacement
TU	Todd units	TVS	transvaginal sonography
	transrectal ultrasound	TVSC	transvaginal sector scan
	tuberculin units	TVU	total volume of urine
TUE	transurethral extraction	TVUS	transvaginal ultrasound
TUF	total ultrafiltration	TW	tapwater
TUIBN	transurethral incision of bladder neck		test weight T-wave
TUIP	transurethral incision of the prostate	TWAR	*Chlamydia psittaci*
TULIP®	transurethral ultrasound-guided laser-induced prostatectomy (system)	T wave	part of the electrocardiographic cycle, representing a portion of ventricular repolarization
TUN	total urinary nitrogen		
TUPR	transurethral prostatic resection	TWD	total white and differential count
TUR	transurethral resection	TWE	tapwater enema
T₃UR	triiodothyronine uptake ratio	TWETC	tapwater enema till clear
		TWG	total weight gain
TURB	turbidity	TWH	transitional wall hyperplasia
TURBN	transurethral resection bladder neck	TWHW ok	toe walking and heel walking all right
TURBT	transurethral resection bladder tumor	TWI	T-wave inversion
TURP	transurethral resection of prostate	TWR	total wrist replacement
		TWWD	tap water wet dressing
TURV	transurethral resection valves	Tx	therapy traction
TUU	transureteroureterostomy		transfuse
TUV	transurethral valve		transplant
TV	television		treatment
	temporary visit		tympanostomy
	tidal volume	T & X	type and crossmatch
	transvenous	TXA₂	thromboxane A₂
	trial visit	TXB₂	thromboxane B₂

176

TXM	type and crossmatch T cell crossmatch		UBC	University of British Columbia (brace)
TYCO #3	Tylenol® with 30 mg of codeine (#1=7.5 mg, #2=15 mg and#4=60 mg of codeine present)		UBF UBI	unknown black female ultraviolet blood irradiation
Tyl	Tylenol® tyloma (callus)		UBM UBO	unknown black male unidentified bright object
TYMP	tympanogram		UBW	usual body weight
TZ	transition zone		UC	ulcerative colitis umbilical cord

U

				unconscious Unit clerk United Church of Christ urea clearance urine culture uterine contraction
U	Ultralente Insulin® units (this is the most dangerous abbreviation —spell out "unit") unknown upper urine		U&C	urethral and cervical usual and customary
			UCD	urine collection device usual childhood diseases
			UCE	urea cycle enzymopathy
			UCG	urinary chorionic gonadotropins
U/1	1 finger breadth below umbilicus		UCHD	usual childhood diseases
1/U	1 finger over umbilicus		UCHS	uncontrolled hemorrhagic shock
U/	at umbilicus		UCI	urethral catheter in
UA	umbilical artery unauthorized absence			usual childhood illnesses
	uncertain about		UCL	uncomfortable loudness level
	upper airway upper arm		UCO	urethral catheter out
	uric acid		UCP	urethral closure pressure
	urinalysis		UCR	unconditioned response
UAC	umbilical artery catheter under active			usual, customary, and reasonable
	upper airway congestion		UCRE	urine creatinine
UAE	urinary albumin excretion		UCRP	universal coagulation reference plasma
UAL	umbilical artery line up *ad lib*		UCS	unconscious
UA&M	urinalysis and microscopy		UCX	urine culture
UAO	upper airway obstruction		UD	as directed urethral dilatation
UAPF	upon arrival patient found			urethral discharge
UAT	up as tolerated			uterine distension
UAVC	univentricular atrioventricular connection		UDC	usual diseases of childhood
			UDCA	ursodeoxycholic acid
			UDN	updraft nebulizer
			UDO	undetermined origin

UDP	unassisted diastolic pressure		immunoelectrophoresis
		UIP	usual interstitial pneumonitis
UDS	unconditioned stimulus	UIQ	upper inner quadrant
UE	under elbow	UJ	universal joint (syndrome)
	undetermined etiology	UK	unknown
	upper extremity		urine potassium
UES	upper esophageal sphincter		urokinase
		UL	Unit Leader
UESP	upper esophageal sphincter pressure		upper left
			upper lid
UF	ultrafiltration	U/L	upper and lower
	until finished	U & L	upper and lower
UFC	urine-free cortisol	ULLE	upper lid, left eye
UFF	unusual facial features	ULN	upper limits of normal
UFFI	urea formaldehyde foam insulation	ULQ	upper left quadrant
		ULRE	upper lid, right eye
UFN	until further notice	ULSB	upper left sternal border
UFO	unflagged order	ULYTES	electrolytes, urine
UFR	ultrafiltration rate	UM	unmarried
UG	until gone	umb ven	umbilical vein
	urinary glucose	UMCD	uremic medullary cystic disease
	urogenital		
UGDP	University Group Diabetes Project	UN	undernourished
			urinary nitrogen
UGH	uveitis, glaucoma, and hyphema (syndrome)	UNA	urinary nitrogen appearance
UGI	upper gastrointestinal series	UNa	urine sodium
		UNC	uncrossed
UGIH	upper gastrointestinal (tract) hemorrhage	unacc	unaccompanied
		ung	ointment
UGK	urine glucose ketones	UNK	unknown
UGP	urinary gonadotropin peptide	UNL	upper normal levels
		UNOS	United Network for Organ Sharing
UH	umbilical hernia		
	University Hospital	UO	under observation
UHBI	upper hemibody irradiation		undetermined origin
			ureteral orifice
UHDDS	Uniform Hospital Discharge Data Set		urinary output
		UOP	urinary output
UHP	University Health Plan	UOQ	upper outer quadrant
UI	urinary incontinence	Uosm	urinary osmolality
UIB	Unemployment Insurance Benefits	✔ up	check up
		UP	unipolar
UIBC	unsaturated iron binding capacity	U/P	urine to plasma (creatinine)
UID	once daily (this is a dangerous abbreviation, spell out "once daily")	UPEP	urine protein electrophoresis
UIEP	urine (urinary)	UPJ	ureteropelvic junction

UPOR	usual place of residence	USOH	usual state of health
UPP	urethral pressure profile	USP	unassisted systolic
UPPP	uvulopalatopharyngo-		pressure
	plasty		United States
U/P ratio	urine to plasma ratio		Pharmacopeia
UPT	uptake	USPHS	United States Public
	urine pregnancy test		Health Service
UR	upper right	USUCVD	unsterile uncontrolled
	urinary retention		vaginal delivery
	utilization review	USVMD	urine specimen volume
URAC	uric acid		measuring device
URD	undifferentiated	UTD	up to date
	respiratory disease	*ut dict*	as directed
URI	upper respiratory infection	UTF	usual throat flora
URIC A	uric acid	UTI	urinary tract infection
url	unrelated	UTO	unable to obtain
URO	urology		upper tibial osteotomy
UROB	urobilinogen	UTS	ulnar tunnel syndrome
urol	urology		ultrasound
URQ	upper right quadrant	UUN	urinary urea nitrogen
URSB	upper right sternal border	UV	ultraviolet
URTI	upper respiratory tract		ureterovesical
	infection		urine volume
US	ultrasonography	UVA	ultraviolet A light
	unit secretary		ureterovesical angle
USA	unit services assistant	UVB	ultraviolet B light
	United States Army	UVC	umbilical vein catheter
	unstable angina	UVJ	ureterovesical junction
USAF	United States Air Force	UVL	ultraviolet light
USAN	United States Adopted		umbilical venous line
	Names	UVR	ultraviolet radiation
USAP	unstable angina pectoris	UVT	unsustained ventricular
USB	upper sternal border		tachycardia
U-SCOPE	ureteroscopy	U/WB	unit of whole blood
USCVD	unsterile controlled	UW	unilateral weakness
	vaginal delivery	UWF	unknown white female
USDA	United States Department	UWM	unknown white male
	of Agriculture		unwed mother
USG	ultrasonography		
USH	United Services for		
	Handicapped		
	usual state of health		
USI	urinary stress		
	incontinence		**V**
USMC	United States Marine		
	Corp		
USN	ultrasonic nebulizer		
	United States Navy	V	five
USOGH	usual state of good health		gas volume

179

	minute volume		bundle electrocardiogram
	vagina		
	vein	VAHRA	ventricular atrial height right atrium
	verb		
	vomiting	VAIN	vaginal intraepithelial neoplasia
$\dot{v}$	ventilation (L/min)		
+V	positive vertical divergence	VALE	visual acuity, left eye
V1	fifth cranial nerve, ophthalmic division	VAMC	Veterans Affairs Medical Center
V2	fifth cranial nerve, maxillary division	VAMS	Visual Analogue Mood Scale
V3	fifth cranial nerve, mandibular division	VANCO/P	vancomycin-peak
		VANCO/T	vancomycin-trough
V_1 to V_6	precordial chest leads	VAOD	visual acuity, right eye
VA	vacuum aspiration	VAOS	visual acuity, left eye
	valproic acid	VA OS LP with P	visual acuity, left eye, left perception with projection
	Veterans Administration		
	visual acuity	VAP	ventilator-associated pneumonia
V_A	alveolar gas volume		
V&A	vagotomy and antrectomy		venous access port
VAB	vinblastine, dactinomycin, bleomycin, cisplatin, and cyclophosphamide		vincristine, asparaginase, and prednisone
		VAPCS	ventricular atrial proximal coronary sinus
VAC	ventriculo-arterial connections	VAR	variant
		VARE	visual acuity, right eye
	vincristine, dactinomycin, and cyclophosphamide	VAS	vascular
			Visual Analogue Scale
	vincristine, doxorubicin, and cyclophosphamide	VASC	Visual-Auditory Screen Test for Children
VAD	vascular (venous) access device	VAS RAD	vascular radiology
		VATER	vertebral, anal, tracheal, esophageal, and renal anomalies
	ventricular assist device		
	Veterans Administration Domiciliary		
		VATH	vinblastine, doxorubicin, thiotepa, and fluoxymesterone
	vincristine, doxorubicin, and dexamethasone		
VADCS	ventricular atrial distal coronary sinus	VB	Van Buren (catheter)
			venous blood
VADRIAC	vincristine, doxorubicin, and cyclophosphamide		vinblastine and methotrexate
VAERS	Vaccine Adverse Events Reporting System	VB_1	first voided bladder specimen
vag.	vagina	VB_2	second midstream bladder specimen
VAG HYST	vaginal hysterectomy	VBAC	vaginal birth after cesarean
VAH	Veterans Administration Hospital		
VAHBE	ventricular atrial His	VBAP	vincristine, carmustine,

	doxorubicin, and prednisone	VDD	atrial synchronous ventricular inhibited pacing
VBC	vinblastine, bleomycin, and cisplatin	VDG	venereal disease—gonorrhea
VBD	vinblastine, bleomycin, and cisplatin	Vdg	voiding
VBG	venous blood gas vertical banded gastroplasty	VDH	valvular disease of the heart
VBI	vertebrobasilar insufficiency	VDL	variable diversity joining vasodepressor lipid visual detection level
VBL	vinblastine	VDO	varus derotational osteotomy
VBP	vinblastine, bleomycin, and cisplatin	VD or M	venous distention or masses
VBS	vertebral-basilar system	VDP	vinblastine, dacarbazine, and cisplatin
VC	color vision etoposide and carboplatin pulmonary capillary blood volume vena cava vital capacity vocal cords	VDRL	Venereal Disease Research Laboratory (test for syphilis)
V&C	vertical and centric (a bite)	VDRR	vitamin D-resistant rickets
VCAP	vincristine, cyclophosphamide, doxorubicin, and prednisone	VDS	venereal disease—syphilis vindesine
		VDT	video display terminal
Vcc	vision with correction	VD/VT	dead space to tidal volume ratio
VCCA	velocity common carotid artery	VE	vaginal examination vertex vocational evaluation
VCG	vectorcardiography	V_E	minute volume (expired)
VCO	ventilator CPAP oxyhood	V/E	violence and eloper
VCR	video cassette recorder vincristine sulfate	VEA	ventricular ectopic activity
VCT	venous clotting time	VEB	ventricular ectopic beat
VCU	voiding cystourethrogram	VEC	vecuronium
VCUG	vesicoureterogram voiding cystourethrogram	VED	vacuum extraction delivery ventricular ectopic depolarization
VD	venereal disease voided volume of distribution	VEE	Venezuelan equine encephalitis
V_D	deadspace volume	VENT	ventilation ventilator ventral ventricular
V_d	volume of distribution		
V&D	vomiting and diarrhea		
VDA	venous digital angiogram visual discriminatory acuity	VEP	visual evoked potential
		VER	ventricular escape rhythm visual evoked responses
VDAC	vaginal delivery after cesarean	VES	ventricular extrasystoles

VET	veteran		vinblastine, ifosfamide, and cisplatin
VF	left leg (electrode)		voluntary interruption of pregnancy
	ventricular fibrillation	VIPomas	vasoactive intestinal peptide-secreting tumors
	vision field		
	vocal fremitus		
VFI	visual fields intact		
V. Fib	ventricular fibrillation		
VFP	vitreous fluorophotometry	VIQ	Verbal Intelligence Quotient (part of Wechsler tests)
VFPN	Volu-feed premie nipple		
VFRN	Volu-feed regular nipple		
VG	vein graft	VIS	Visual Impairment Service
	ventricular gallop		
	very good	VISC	vitreous infusion suction cutter
V&G	vagotomy and gastroenterotomy		
		VISI	volar intercalated segmental instability
VGH	very good health		
VH	vaginal hysterectomy	VIT	venom immunotherapy
	Veterans Hospital		vital
	viral hepatitis		vitamin
	vitreous hemorrhage	vit. cap.	vital capacity
	von Herrick (grading system)	VIU	visual internal urethrotomy
VH I	very narrow anterior chamber angles	VIZ	namely
		V-J	ventriculo-jugular (shunt)
VH II	moderately narrow anterior chamber angles	VKC	vernal keratoconjunctivitis
		VKH	Vogt-Koyanagi-Harada's disease
VH III	moderately wide open anterior chamber angles		
		VL	left arm (electrode)
VH IV	wide open anterior chamber angles		vial
		VLBW	very low birth weight
VHD	valvular heart disease	VLCD	very low calorie diet
VI	six	VLCFA	very long chain fatty acids
	volume index		
vib	vibration	VLDL	very low density lipoprotein
VIBS	Victim's Information Bureau Service		
		VLH	ventrolateral nucleus of the hypothalamus
VICA	velocity internal carotid artery		
		VLM	visceral larva migrans
VID	videodensitometry	VLP	virus like particle
VIG	vaccinia immune globulin	VLR	vastus lateralis release
VIN	vulvar intraepithelial neoplasm	VM	ventilated mask
			ventimask
VIP	etopside, ifosfamide, and cisplatin		Venturi mask
			vestibular membrane
	vasoactive intestinal peptide	VM 26	teniposide
		VMA	vanillylmandelic acid
	vasoactive intracorporeal pharmacotherapy	VMCP	vincristine, melphalan, cyclophosphamide, and prednisone
	very important patient		

VMH	ventromedial hypothalamus	VQ	ventilation perfusion
VMO	vastus medalis oblique	VR	valve replacement
VMR	vasomotor rhinitis		right arm (electrode)
VN	visiting nurse		ventricular rhythm
VNA	Visiting Nurses' Association		verbal reprimand
			vocational rehabilitation
VNC	vesicle neck contracture	VRA	visual reinforcement audiometry
VO	verbal order	VRC	vocational rehabilitation counselor
VO$_2$	oxygen consumption		
VOCAB	vocabulary	VRI	viral respiratory infection
VOCTOR	void on call to operating room	VRL	ventral root, lumbar
		VRT	variance of resident time
VOD	veno-occlusive disease		ventral root, thoracic
	vision right eye		vertical radiation topography
VOL	volume		
	voluntary		Visual Retention Test
VOM	vomited	VRU	ventilator rehabilitation unit
VOO	continuous ventricular asynchronous pacing	VS	vagal stimulation
			versus
VOR	vestibular ocular reflex		very sensitive
VOS	vision left eye		visited
VOT	Visual Organization Test		vital signs (temperature, pulse, and respiration)
VOU	vision both eyes		
VP	etoposide	VSBE	very short below elbow (cast)
	variegate porphyria		
	venipuncture	VSD	ventricular septal defect
	venous pressure	VSI	visual motor integration
	ventriculo-peritoneal	VSN	vital signs normal
V & P	vagotomy and pyloroplasty	VSO	vertical subcondylar oblique
	ventilation and perfusion	VSOK	vital signs normal
VP-16	etoposide	VSR	venous stasis retinopathy
VPA	valproic acid	VSS	vital signs stable
V-Pad	sanitary napkin	V$_{ss}$	apparent volume of distribution
VPB	ventricular premature beat		
VPC	ventricular premature contractions	VSSAF	vital signs stable, afebrile
		VSV	vesicular stomatitis virus
VPDF	vegetable protein diet plus fiber	VT	validation therapy
			ventricular tachycardia
VPDs	ventricular premature depolarizations	V$_t$	tidal volume
		v. tach.	ventricular tachycardia
VPI	velopharyngeal incompetence	VTE	venous thromboembolism
		VTEC	verotoxin-producing *Escherichia coli*
	velopharyngeal insufficiency		
VPL	ventro-posterolateral	VT-NS	ventricular tachycardia non-sustained
VPR	volume pressure response	VTP	voluntary termination of pregnancy
VPS	valvular pulmonic stenosis		

VT-S	ventricular tachycardia sustained	W or A	weakness or atrophy
		WAF	weakness, atrophy, and fasciculation
VT/VF	ventricular tachycardia/fibrillation		white adult female
VTX	vertex	WAIS	Wechsler Adult Intelligence Scale
VUR	vesicoureteral reflux		
VV	varicose veins	WAIS-R	Wechsler Adult Intelligence Scale-Revised
V&V	vulva and vagina		
V/V	volume to volume ratio		
VVC	vulvovaginal candidiasis	WAM	white adult male
VVD	vaginal vertex delivery	WAP	wandering atrial pacemaker
VVFR	vesicovaginal fistula repair		
		WAS	Wiskott-Aldrich syndrome
V/VI	grade 5 on a 6 grade basis	WASO	wakefulness after sleep onset
VVI	ventricular demand pacing	WASS	Wasserman test
VVOR	visual-vestibulo-ocular-reflex	WAT	word association test
		WB	waist belt
VVT	ventricular synchronous pacing		weight bearing
			well baby
VW	vessel wall		Western blot
VWD	von Willebrand's disease		whole blood
vWF	von Willebrand factor	WBACT	whole blood activated clotting time
VWM	ventricular wall motion		
V_x	vitrectomy	WBAT	weight bearing as tolerated
V-XT	V-pattern exotropia		
VZ	varicella zoster	WBC	well baby clinic
VZIG	varicella zoster immune globulin		white blood cell (count)
		WBCT	whole blood clotting time
VZV	varicella zoster virus	WBH	whole-body hyperthermia
		W Bld	whole blood
		WBN	wellborn nursery
		WBPTT	whole blood partial thromboplastin time

W

		WBQC	wide base quad cane
		WBR	whole body radiation
		WBS	whole body scan
		WBTF	Waring Blender tube feeding
W	wearing glasses	
	week	WBTT	weight bearing to tolerance
	weight	
	well	WBUS	weeks by ultrasound
	white	WC	ward clerk
	widowed		ward confinement
	wife		warm compress
	with		wet compresses
WA	when awake		wheelchair
	while awake		when called
	wide awake		white count

	whooping cough	WFR	wheel-and-flare reaction
	will call	WH	walking heel (cast)
WCA	work capacity assessment		well hydrated
WCC	well child care	WHO	World Health
	white cell count		Organization
WCM	whole cow's milk		wrist-hand orthosis
WCS	work capacity specialist	WHPB	whirlpool bath
WD	ward	WHV	woodchuck hepatitis virus
	well developed	WHVP	wedged hepatic venous
	well differentiated		pressure
	wet dressing	WHZ	wheezes
	Wilson's disease	WI	ventricular demand pacing
	word		walk-in
	wound	W/I	within
W/D	warm and dry	W+I	work and interest
	withdrawal	WIA	wounded in action
W→D	wet to dry	WIC	women, infants, and
W4D	Worth four-dot (test for		children
	fusion)	WID	widow
WDCC	well-developed collateral		widower
	circulation	WIS	Ward Incapacity Scale
WDF	white divorced female	WISC	Wechsler Intelligence
WDHA	watery diarrhea,		Scale for Children
	hypokalemia, and	WISC-R	Wechsler Intelligence
	achlorhydria		Scale for Children-
WDHH	watery diarrhea,		Revised
	hypokalemia, and	wk	week
	hypochlorhydria	WKI	Wakefield Inventory
WDLL	well-differentiated	WL	waiting list
	lymphocytic lymphoma		weight loss
WDM	white divorced male	WLS	wet lung syndrome
WDWN-BM	well-developed,	WLT	waterload test
	well-nourished black	WK	week
	male		work
WDWN-WF	well-developed,	WKS	Wernicke-Korsakoff
	well-nourished white		syndrome
	female	WM	white male
WE	weekend	WMA	wall motion abnormality
W/E	weekend	WMD	warm moist dressings
WEE	Western equine		(sterile)
	encephalitis	WMF	white married female
WEP	weekend pass	WMI	wall motion index
WF	white female	WMM	white married male
W FEEDS	with feedings	WMP	warm moist packs (unsterile)
WFH	white-faced hornet		weight management
WFI	water for injection		program
WFL	within full limits	WMS	Wechsler Memory Scale
	within functional limits	WMX	whirlpool, massage, and
WF-O	will follow in office		exercise

WN	well nourished		weight (wt)
WND	wound		Wilms' tumor
WNL	within normal limits		wisdom teeth
WNLS	weighted nonlinear least squares	W-T-D	wet to dry
WNt^{50}	Wagner-Nelson time 50 hours	WTS	whole tomography slice
		W/U	workup
WO	weeks old	WV	whispered voice
	written order	W/V	weight-to-volume ratio
W/O	water in oil	WW	Weight Watchers
	without	W/W	weight-to-weight ratio
WOB	work of breathing	W→W	wet to wet
WOP	without pain	WWAC	walk with aid of cane
W.P.	whirlpool	WWidF	white widowed female
WPCs	washed packed cells	WWidM	white widowed male
WPFM	Wright peak flow meter	WYOU	women years of usage
WPOA	wearing patch on arrival		
WPP	Wechsler Preschool Primary Scale of Intelligence		
WPPSI	Wechsler Preschool Primary Scale of Intelligence		

X

WPPSI-R	WPPSI revised		
WPW	Wolff-Parkinson-White (syndrome)	X	break
			cross
WR	Wassermann reaction		crossmatch
	wrist		except
WRAT	Wide Range Achievement Test		exophoria for distance
			start of anesthesia
WRAT-R	The Wide Range Achievement Test, Revised		ten
			times
			xylocaine
WRBC	washed red blood cells	X′	exophoria for near
WRC	washed red (blood) cells	X	except
WRIOT	Wide Range Interest-Opinion Test (for career planning)	X^2	chi-square
		X+#	xyphoid plus number of fingerbreadths
WS	ward secretary	X3	orientation as to time, place and person
	watt seconds		
	work simplification	XBT	xylose breath test
	work simulation	XC	excretory cystogram
W&S	wound and skin	XD	times daily
WSepF	white separated female	X&D	examination and diagnosis
WSepM	white separated male	X2d	times two days
WSF	white single female	XDP	xeroderma pigmentosum
WSM	white single male	Xe	xenon
WSP	wearable speech processor	XeCT	xenon-enhanced computed tomography
WT	walking tank		

X-ed	crossed			**Y**
XFER	transfer			
XGP	xanthogranulomatous pyelonephritis			
XI	eleven			
XII	twelve	YACP	young adult chronic patient	
XIP	x-ray in plaster			
XKO	not knocked out	YAG	yttrium aluminum garnet (laser)	
XL	extended release (once a day oral solid dosage form)	Yb	ytterbium	
	extra large	YBOCS	Yale-Brown Obsessive-Compulsive Scale	
XLA	X-linked infantile agammaglobulinemia			
		Yel	yellow	
X-leg	cross leg	YF	yellow fever	
XLH	X-linked hypophos-phatemia	YFH	yellow-faced hornet	
		YFI	yellow fever immunization	
XLJR	X-linked juvenile retinoschisis			
		YJV	yellow jacket venom	
XM	crossmatch	YLC	youngest living child	
X-mat.	crossmatch	YMC	young male Caucasian	
XMM	xeromammography	Y/N	yes/no	
XOM	extraocular movements	YO	years old	
XOP	x-ray out of plaster	YOB	year of birth	
XP	xeroderma pigmentosum	YORA	younger-onset rheumatoid arthritis	
XR	x-ray			
XRT	radiation therapy	YPLL	years of potential life lost before age 65	
XS	excessive			
XS-LIM	exceeds limits of procedure	yr	year	
		YSC	yolk sac carcinoma	
XT	exotropia	YTD	year to date	
X(T)	intermittent exotropia	YTDY	yesterday	
XU	excretory urogram			
XULN	times upper limit of normal			
XV	fifteen			
3X/WK	three times a week			**Z**
XX	normal female sex chromosome type			
	twenty			
XX/XY	sex karyotypes	Z	impedance	
XXX	thirty	ZDV	zidovudine	
XY	normal male sex chromosome type	Z-E	Zollinger-Ellison (syndrome)	
XYL	Xylocaine®	ZEEP	zero end-expiratory pressure	
XYLO	Xylocaine®	ZES	Zollinger-Ellison syndrome	

Z-ESR	zeta erythrocyte sedimentation rate	ZnOE	zinc oxide and eugenol
ZIG	zoster serum immune globulin	ZNS	zonisamide
		ZPC	zero point of charge
			zopiclone
ZIP	zoster immune plasma	ZPO	zinc peroxide
ZMC	zygomatic	ZPP	zinc protoporphyrin
	zygomatic maxillary compound (complex)	ZPT	zinc pyrithione
		ZSB	zero stools since birth
Zn	zinc	ZSR	zeta sedimentation rate
ZnO	zinc oxide		

Symbols and Numbers

↑	above
	alive
	elevated
	greater than
	high
	improved
	increase
	rising
	up
↓	dead
	decrease
	depressed
	down
	falling
	lowered
	normal plantar reflex
	restricted
→	causes to
	greater than
	progressing
	results in
	showed
	to the right
	transfer to
←	less than
	resulted from
	to the left
↔	same as
	stable
	to and from
	unchanging
↓↓	flexor
	testes descended
↑↑	extensor
	positive Babinsky
	testes undescended
||	parallel
	parallel bars
✓	check
	flexion
#	fracture
	number
	pound
∴	therefore
Δ scan	delta scan (computed tomography scan)
+	plus
	positive
	present
−	absent
	minus
	negative
/	slash mark signifying per, and, or with (this is a dangerous symbol as it is mistaken for a one)
±	either positive or negative
	no definite cause
	plus or minus
	very slight trace
⌐	right lower quadrant
⌐	right upper quadrant
⌐	left upper quadrant
⌐	left lower quadrant
>	greater than
	left ear-bone conduction threshold
≥	greater than or equal to
<	caused by
	less than
	right ear-bone conduction threshold
≤	less than or equal to
⋪	not less than
⋫	not more than
∧	above
	diastolic blood pressure
	increased
∨	below
	systolic blood pressure
≠	not equal to
≅	approximately equal to
≈	approximately
×	left ear-air conduction threshold
	ten

]	left ear-masked bone conduction threshold	□	living male left ear-masked air conduction threshold
△	right ear-masked air conduction threshold	○	living female right ear-bone conduction threshold
[	right ear-masked bone conduction threshold	◇	sex unknown
⊖	reversible	(□)	adopted living male
?	questionable	*	birth
∅	no none	†	dead death
@	at		
1°	first degree primary	♀	standing
1:1	one-to-one (individual session with staff)	o—<	recumbent position
2°	second degree secondary	♂ (sitting)	sitting position
3°	tertiary third degree	♥	heart
24°	twenty-four hours	A α	alpha
777	Ortho Novum 777® (a triphasic oral contraceptive)	B β	beta
		Γ γ	gamma
		Δ δ	anion gap
i	one (Roman numerals are dangerous expressions and should not be used)		change
			delta
			delta gap
			prism diopter
			temperature
			trimester
ii	two		
iii	three	E ε	epsilon
iiii	four	Z ζ	zeta
iv	four (this is a dangerous abbreviation as it is read as intravenous, use 4)	H η	eta
		Θ θ	negative theta
		I ι	iota
		K κ	kappa
		Λ λ	lambda
v	five	M μ	micro mu
vi	six		
vii	seven	N ν	nu
viii	eight	Ξ ξ	xi
ix	nine	O o	omicron
x	ten	Π π	pi
xi	eleven	P ρ	rho
xii	twelve	Σ σ	sigma sum of summary
♂	male		
♀	female	T τ	tau
■	deceased male	Υ υ	upsilon
●	deceased female		

Φ φ	phenyl	"	inches
	phi		seconds
	thyroid	⊙	start of an operation
X χ	chi	⊗	end of anesthesia
Ψ ψ	psi	3×	three times
	psychiatric	2×2	gauze dressing
			folded 2″ x 2″
Ω ω	omega		
′	feet	4×4	gauze dressing
	minutes (as in 30′)		folded 4″ x 4″

Numbers for teeth

1	upper right 3rd molar	17	lower left 3rd molar
2	upper right 2nd molar	18	lower left 2nd molar
3	upper right 1st molar	19	lower left 1st molar
4	upper right 2nd bicuspid	20	lower left 2nd bicuspid
5	upper right 1st bicuspid	21	lower left 1st bicuspid
6	upper right canine (eyetooth)	22	lower left canine
7	upper right lateral incisor	23	lower left lateral incisor
8	upper right central incisor	24	lower left central incisor
9	upper left central incisor	25	lower right central incisor
10	upper left lateral incisor	26	lower right lateral incisor
11	upper left canine	27	lower right canine
12	upper left 1st bicuspid	28	lower right 1st bicuspid
13	upper left 2nd bicuspid	29	lower right 2nd bicuspid
14	upper left 1st molar	30	lower right 1st molar
15	upper left 2nd molar	31	lower right 2nd molar
16	upper left 3rd molar	32	lower right 3rd molar

Shorthand for laboratory test values

See text for meaning of the abbreviations shown

Complete Blood Count

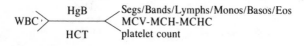

WBC⟩ HgB ⟨ Segs/Bands/Lymphs/Monos/Basos/Eos
       HCT   MCV-MCH-MCHC
             platelet count

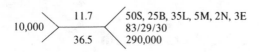

10,000 ⟩ 11.7 ⟨ 50S, 25B, 35L, 5M, 2N, 3E
         36.5   83/29/30
                290,000

Electrolytes

sodium	chloride
potassium	bicarbonate

142	99
4.7	25

SMA 6 (Astra 7)

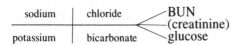

sodium	chloride
potassium	bicarbonate

⟨ BUN
  (creatinine)
  glucose

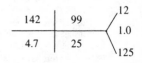

142	99
4.7	25

⟨ 12
  1.0
  125

Blood Gases
7.4/80/48/98/25   pH/PO₂/PCO₂/% O₂ Saturation/bicarbonate

Obstetrical shorthand

$\dfrac{2 \text{ cm} | 80\%}{-2 \text{ Vtx}}$ 2 cm = dilation of cervix

80% = degree of cer-
  vix effacement
Vtx = vertex; presen-
  tation of fetus,
(breech = Br)

−2=station; distance
  above (−) or
  below (+) the
  spine of the
  ischium
  measured in cm

Reflexes[6]

Reflexes are usually graded on a 0 to 4+ scale:

4+   may indicate disease
     often associated with clonus
     very brisk, hyperactive (or ++++)
3+   brisker than average
     possibly but not necessarily indicative of disease
       (or +++)
2+   average
     normal (or ++)
1+   low normal
     somewhat diminished (or +)
0   may indicate neuropathy
     no response

Muscle strength[6]

0—No muscular contraction detected
1—A barely detectable flicker or trace of contraction
2—Active movement of the body part with gravity eliminated
3—Active movement against gravity
4—Active movement against gravity and some resistance
5—Active movement against full resistance without evident
   fatigue. This is normal muscle strength

Pulse[6]

 0   completely absent
+1   markedly impaired (or 1+, or +)
+2   moderately impaired (or 2+, or ++)
+3   slightly impaired (or 3+, or +++)
+4   normal (or 4+, or ++++)

Gradation of intensity of heart murmurs[6]

1/6 or I/VI   may not be heard in all positions
                 very faint, heard only after the listener has
                   "tuned in"

2/6 or II/VI	quiet, but heard immediately upon placing the stethoscope on the chest
3/6 or III/VI	moderately loud
4/6 or IV/VI	loud
5/6 or V/VI	very loud, may be heard with a stethoscope partly off the chest (thrills are associated)
6/6 or VI/VI	may be heard with the stethoscope entirely off the chest (thrills are associated)

Apothecary symbols

The symbols presented below are for informational use. The apothecary system should *not* be used. Only the metric system should be used. The methods of expressing the symbols, the meanings, and the equivalences are not the classic ones, nor are they accurate, but reflect the usual intended meanings when used by some older physicians in writing prescription directions.

ℨ or ℨ͐	dram, teaspoonful, (5 mL)	℥ or ℥i		ounce, (30 mL)
		gr		grain (approximately 60 mg)
ℨii	two drams, 2 teaspoonfuls, (10 mL)			
		ℳ		minim (approximately 0.06 mL)
℥ss	half ounce, tablespoonful, (15 mL)	gtt		drop

References

1. CBE Style Manual, 5th ed. Bethesda, MD: Council of Biology Editors; 1983.

2. Gennaro AR, ed. Remington's Pharmaceutical Sciences, 18th ed. Easton, PA: Mack Publishing Co; 1990; 1831.

3. Davis NM, Cohen MR. Medication errors: causes and prevention. Huntingdon Valley, PA: Neil M. Davis Associates; 1983.

4. Cohen MR. Medication error reports. Hosp Pharm (appears monthly from 1975 to the present).

5. Cohen MR. Medication errors. Nursing 93 (appears monthly, starting in Nursing 77, to the present).

6. Bates B. A guide to physical examinations and history taking, 5th ed. Philadelphia: J.B. Lippincott; 1991.

Please forward additional meanings for these abbreviations, additional abbreviations and their meanings, or corrections to the author so that the list can be updated. Thank you. Dr. Neil M. Davis, 1143 Wright Drive, Huntingdon Valley, PA 19006. FAX (215) 938 1937

Normal Laboratory Values*

In the following tables, normal reference values for commonly requested laboratory tests are listed in traditional units and in SI units. The tables are a guideline only. Values are method dependent and "normal values" may vary between laboratories.

Blood, Plasma or Serum		
Determination	**Reference Value**	
	Conventional Units	**SI Units**
Ammonia	10–80 μg/dl	5–50 μmol/L
Amylase	0–130 units/L	0–130 units/L
Antinuclear antibodies	negative at 1:8 dilution of serum	
Bilirubin: direct	≤ 0.2 mg/dl	≤ 4 μmol/L
total	0.1–1 mg/dl	2–18 μmol/L
Calcitonin, male	0–14 pg/mL	0–4.1 pmol/L
female	0–28 pg/mL	0–8.2 pmol/L
medullary carcinoma	>100 pg/mL	>29.3 pmol/L
Calcium[1]	8.8–10.3 mg/dl	2.2–2.6 mmol/L
Carbon dioxide content	22–28 mEq/L	22–28 mmol/L
Chloride	95–105 mEq/L	95–105 mmol/L
Coagulation screen:		
Bleeding time	3–9.5 min	180–570 sec
Prothrombin time	< 2 sec from control	< 2 sec from control
Partial thromboplastin time activated	25–38 sec	25–38 sec
Copper, total	70–140 μg/dl	11–22 μmol/L
Corticotropin (ACTH)	20–100 pg/mL	4–22 pmol/L
Cortisol: 8 am	5–25 μg/dl	0.14–0.69 μmol/L
8 pm	< 10 μg/dl	< 0.28 μmol/L
4 hr ACTH test	30–45 μg/dl	0.83–1.24 μmol/L
Overnight suppression test	< 5 μg/dl	< 0.14 μmol/L
Creatine phosphokinase, total (CK, CPK)	≤ 130 units/L	≤ 130 units/L
Creatine phosphokinase isoenzymes	CK-MB = ≤ 5% total CK	≤ 0.05
Creatinine	0.6–1.2 mg/dl	50–100 μmol/L
Follicle stimulating hormone (FSH):		2–15 IU/L
female	2–15 mIU/mL	20–50 IU/L
peak production	20–50 mIU/ mL	1–10 IU/L
male	1–10 mIU/mL	
Glucose fasting	70–110 mg/dl	3.9–6.1 mmol/L
Hematologic tests:		
Hematocrit (Hct), female	33%–43%	0.33–0.43
male	39%–49%	0.39–0.49
Hemoglobin (Hb), female	11.5–15.5 g/dl	115–155 g/L
male	14–18 g/dl	140–180 g/L
Leukocyte count (WBC)	3200–9800/mm³	3.2–9.8 × 10⁹/L
Erythrocyte count (RBC), female	3.5–5 million/mm³	3.5–5 × 10¹²/L
male	4.3–5.9 million/mm³	4.3–5.9 × 10¹²/L
Mean corpuscular volume (MCV)	76–100 μm³/cell	76–100 fl/cell
Mean corpuscular hemoglobin (MCH)	27–33 pg/RBC	27–33 pg/RBC
Mean corpuscular hemoglobin concentration (MCHC)	33–37 g/dl	330–370 g/L

[1] Slightly higher in children
* ©1992 by Facts and Comparisons. Used with permission from *Drug Facts and Comparisons, 1992 ed.* St. Louis: Facts and Comparisons, a Division of the J.B. Lippincott Company.

Normal Laboratory Values (Cont.)

	Blood, Plasma or Serum (Cont.)	
	Reference Value	
Determination	**Conventional Units**	**SI Units**
Hematologic tests (cont.):		
Erythrocyte sedimentation rate		
(sedrate, ESR): female	≤ 30 mm/hr	≤ 30 mm/hr
male	≤ 20 mm/hr	≤ 20 mm/hr
Erythrocyte enzymes:		
Glucose-6-phosphate dehydrogenase		
(G6PD)	5–15 units/g Hb	5–15 units/g Hb
Pyruvate kinase	13–17 units/g Hb	13–17 units/g Hb
Ferritin (serum): Iron deficiency	0–12 ng/mL	0–4.8 nmol/L
Borderline	13–20 ng/mL	5.2–8 nmol/L
Iron excess	> 400 ng/L	> 160 nmol/L
Folic acid: normal	>3.3 ng/mL	> 7.3 nmol/L
borderline	2.5–3.2 ng/mL	5.75–7.39 nmol/L
Platelet count	150,000–450,000/mm³	150–450 × 10⁹/L
Vitamin B₁₂: normal	205–876 pg/mL	150–674 pmol/L
borderline	140–204 pg/mL	102.6–149 pmol/L
Iron		
female	60–160 μg/dl	11–29 μmol/L
male	80–180 μg/dl	14–32 μmol/L
Iron binding capacity	250–460 μg/dl	45–82 μmol/L
Lactic acid	0.5–2.2 mmol/L	0.5–2.2 mmol/L
Lactic dehydrogenase	50–150 units/L	50–150 units/L
Lead	≤ 50 μg/dl	≤ 2.4 μmol/L
Lipids: Cholesterol		
< 29 yr	< 200 mg/dl	< 5.2 mmol/L
30–39 yr	< 225 mg/dl	< 5.85 mmol/L
40–49 yr	< 245 mg/dl	< 6.35 mmol/L
> 50 yr	< 265 mg/dl	< 6.85 mmol/L
Triglycerides	40–150 mg/dl	0.4–1.5 g/L
LDL	50–190 mg/dl	1.3–4.9 mmol/L
HDL		
female	30–90 mg/dl	0.8–2.35 mmol/L
male	30–70 mg/dl	0.8–1.8 mmol/L
Magnesium	1.8–3 mEq/L	0.8–1.2 mmol/L
Osmolality	280–296 mOsm/kg water	280–296 mmol/kg
Oxygen saturation (arterial)	96%–100%	0.96–1
PCO₂, Arterial	35–45 mm Hg	4.7–6 kPa
pH, Arterial	7.35–7.45	7.35–7.45
PO₂, Arterial: breathing room air[1]	75–100 mm Hg	10–13.3 kPa
on 100% O₂	> 500 mm Hg	
Phosphatase (acid), total:	≤ 3 King-Armstrong units/dl	≤ 5.5 units/L
	≤ 3 Bodansky units/dl	≤ 16.1 units/L
Phosphatase (alkaline)[2]	30–120 units/L	30–120 units/L
Phosphorus, inorganic[3]	2.5–5 mg/dl	0.8–1.6 mmol/L
Potassium	3.5–5 mEq/L	3.5–5 mmol/L

[1] Age dependent.
[2] Infants and adolescents up to 104 units/L.
[3] Infants in the first year up to 6 mg/dl.

Blood, Plasma or Serum (Cont.)		
	Reference Value	
Determination	**Conventional Units**	**SI Units**
Progesterone Follicular phase Luteal phase	< 2 ng/mL 2–20 ng/mL	< 6 nmol/L 6–64 nmol/L
Prolactin	2–15 ng/mL	0.08–6 nmol/L
Protein: Total Albumin Globulin	6–8 g/dl 4–6 g/dl 2.3–3.5 g/dl	60–80 g/L 40–60 g/L 23–35 g/L
Rheumatoid factor	< 60 IU/mL	
Sodium	135–147 mEq/L	135–147 mmol/L
Testosterone: female male	< 0.6 ng/mL 4–8 ng/mL	< 2 nmol/L 14–28 nmol/L
Thyroid Hormone Function Tests: Thyroid-stimulating hormone (TSH) Thyroxine-binding globulin capacity Total triiodothyronine (T_3) Total thyroxine by RIA (T_4) T_3 resin uptake	0.5–5 μ units/mL 15–25 μg T_4/dl 75–220 ng/dl 4–12 μg/dl 25%–35%	0.5–5 arb unit 193–322 nmol/L 1.2–3.4 nmol/L 52–154 nmol/L 0.25–0.35
Transaminase, AST (Aspartate aminotransferase, SGOT)	≤ 35 units/L	≤ 35 units/L
Transaminase, ALT (Alanine aminotransferase, SGPT)	≤35 units/L	≤ 35 units/L
Urea nitrogen (BUN)	8–18 mg/dl	3–6.5 mmol/L
Uric acid	2–7 mg/dl	120–420 μmol/L
Vitamin A	0.15–0.6 μg/mL	0.5–2.1 μmol/L
Zinc	75–120 μg/dl	11.5–18.5 μmol/L

URINE				
	Reference Value			
Determination	**Conventional Units**		**SI Units**	
Catecholamines: Epinephrine Norepinephrine	< 20 μg/day < 100 μg/day		< 109 nmol/day < 590 nmol/day	
Creatinine	15–25 mg/kg/day		0.13–0.22 mmol/kg/day	
Potassium[1]	25–125 mEq/day		25–125 mmol/day	
Protein, quantitative	< 150 mg/day		< 0.15 g/day	
Sodium[1]	40–220 mEq/day		40–220 mmol/day	

Steroids:	Age (yrs)	(mg/day) male	female	(μmol/day) male	female
17-Ketosteroids	10	1–4	1–4	3–14	3–14
	20	6–21	4–16	21–73	14–56
	30	8–26	4–14	28–90	14–49
	50	5–18	3–9	17–62	10–31
	70	2–10	1–7	7–35	3–24
17-Hydroxycorticosteroids (as cortisol): female male		2–8 mg/day 3–10 mg/day		5–25 μmol/day 10–30 μmol/day	

[1]Varies with intake.

Please forward additional meanings for these abbreviations, additional abbreviations and their meanings, or corrections to the author so that the list can be updated. Thank you. Dr. Neil M. Davis, 1143 Wright Drive, Huntingdon Valley, PA 19006. FAX (215) 938 1937

Additions

_____

_____

_____

_____

_____

_____

_____

_____

_____

_____

_____

_____

_____

_____

_____

_____

_____

_____

_____

_____

_____

_____

Additions

Additions

Additions

Additions

Additions

_____
_____
_____
_____
_____
_____
_____
_____
_____
_____
_____
_____
_____
_____
_____
_____
_____
_____
_____
_____
_____
_____
_____
_____
_____

PRICES

1-4 copies $11.95 each when check or money order **accompanies** the order.

1-4 copies $11.95 each PLUS a $2.00 invoicing fee *per order* to cover the cost of invoicing if payment is not included.

5-19 copies $11.95 each, NO invoicing fee. Purchase order accepted.

20 or more $8.60 each, NO invoicing fee. Purchase order accepted.

United States—Postage cost is included in the price. Pennsylvania residents add 6% sales tax.

Outside of the United States—Prices as shown above plus postage (6.5 ounces or 185 g each). Pay in U.S. dollars through a correspondent U.S. bank.

Make check payable to: Neil M. Davis Associates

Order from: Neil M. Davis Associates
1143 Wright Drive
Huntingdon Valley, PA 19006

Phone (215) 947-1752
FAX (215) 938-1937

ISBN 0-931431-06-9